This book is dedicated to

Marion Jaye Paul,
Lauren Frances Paul
and the memory of
Herbert Lloyd Paul

Before We Were Young

An Exploration of Primordial States of Mind

Michael Ian Paul, MD

esf PUBLISHERS
BINGHAMTON & CLUJ

Published by *Esf* Publishers
1 Marine Midland Plaza
Binghamton, New York 13901, USA
First published 1997

Jacket illustration: Rico Lebrun, *Untitled*, "Dante's Inferno Series," 1962, ink wash on paper. Courtesy of the Estate of Rico Lebrun and Koplin Gallery, Los Angeles, CA.

Author's photograph by Steven Kahn.

Set in Stempl Garamond 10.5/10 pt., and designed by *Esf* Publishers, Binghamton, New York. Printed in the United States of America on acid-free paper.

The paper in this book meets the guidelines for permanence and durability of the Committee on Production Guidelines for Book Longevity of the Council on Library Resources. ∞

ISBN 1-883881-24-2

Table of Contents

Forward by James S. Grotstein 9

Acknowledgments 13

Chapter 1 Introduction 17

Chapter 2 The Sense of Strangeness 29

Chapter 3 A Contribution to the Study of Dimension 39

Chapter 4 A Mental Atlas of the Process of Psychological Birth 59

Chapter 5 Primordial Development of the Penitential Transference 81

Chapter 6 Studies on the Phenomenology of Mental Pressure 107

Chapter 7 Practical Psychoanalytic Epistemology 129

Chapter 8 Intonational Elements as Communication in Psychoanalysis 147

Chapter 9 On the Imitation of Human Speech 165

Chapter 10 Transformational Aspects of Phantasy in Relation to Dyadic Communication Under the Influence of Marijuana 193

References 211

Index 215

Forward

Dr. Paul offers this work as a scientific contribution in which he seeks to establish the emotional coordinates of humanness of the individual patient in this consulting room. In other words, he is approaching the intimacy of the clinical situation with a scientific rigor that borrows of a new perspective of science, one that is post-positivistic, not exclusively dependent on sense data and repeatability and replicability, one that is dependent on questioning the very senses that sense the data of one's encounters, in short an "intuitionistic science," to employ a term from Bion.

Dr. Paul is no stranger to positivistic science. He spent many years as a well-known researcher in molecular pharmacology and neurobio-chemistry in the laboratories of the Brain Research Institute of the UCLA School of Medicine and the National Institute of Health (NIH) in Bethesda, Maryland. He supplemented this rigorous background with yet another rigor, that of psychoanalytic training that ultimately carried him to the psychoanalytic couch of Wilfred Bion, with whom he had also engaged in a clinical research project at UCLA prior to his analysis with him. As if that was not enough, he is also a gifted pianist, dedicated musician, and accomplished sculptor.

This present work, consequently, represents a convergence of Dr. Paul's unique background with neuroscience, art, esthetics, psychoanalytic practice, tutorial and psychoanalytic experience with Bion, and his unique harvesting of the above in the domain of psychoanalytic observation and intuition.

Having been influenced by Bion, Dr. Paul carefully follows one of his prime precepts, that of "abandoning memory, desire, preconceptions, and understanding" so that his sense organs for observation, including intuition, will then, and only then, be unsaturated enough to be capable of "scientific" observations of the patient's emotional life. One of the most perplexing questions in human development, and in the psychoanalytic enterprise as well, is how do we know what we know, and, conjoined with it, how do we develop from what we have learned? These are questions that Bion posed and, in so posing, became the first true epistemologist in psychoanalysis. I have confidence that the readers of Dr. Paul's work will agree with me that the entirety of the unique camera angles he employs in the following chapters constitutes an epistemological foray into the very hardware of psychoanalytic science—in the spirit of Bion yet with his own creative imagination. In his "Introduction" he states the following:

> The point at which pictorial thought translates to verbal thought is a locus of a problem which is very significant—the difference . . . between thought and hallucination. One of the most basic ideas which can be clinically verified is the "simple" notion that translating experience to verbal thought intensifies affect, often to very painful degrees, which initiates attacks on linking (p. 20).

This quotation follows a prefatory remark about the importance of speech and verbal thought. The significance that I read into these remarks was that the infant is born as a bundle of incompletely connected sensory modalities, each of which independently apprehends the needed object(s). How these sense organs begin to cooperate with one another or fail to is far more complex than conventional infant development research on "cross-modality" indicates. If, for instance, one sensory modality (e.g., visualization) is associated with the mother and another sense modality (e.g., audition) with the father, and if the distressed infant or child unconsciously destructively dissociates the linkage between the two, then the ultimate result can be the concretization of that sensory dissociation as a learning disorder. In another chapter, Dr. Paul explores the very essence of the auditory connection between analyst and analysand. Here his background in art and music is invaluable. He highlights the *prosodic* qualities of speech, such as rhythm, intonation, inflection, and timbre. He effectively demonstrates that these dimensions of speech are effective gauges of the authenticity —or lack thereof—of the analysand's ontological status vis à vis the analysis and analyst. Prosodic variants have the capacity to *induce altered states of mind* in the object and thus set up barriers and resistances.

Elsewhere, he explores the clinical significance of certain words which he believes comprise a syndrome of constantly conjoined meanings. These words include *weird*, *strange*, *stupid*, and *dumb*. He reviews the primal meanings of these words and shows how these primal affect-laden meanings persist in their later common usages. He relates these words to different stages of emergence from states of projective identification into states of separateness. *Dumb* represents the mental quality that obtains when the analysand is in the state of projective identification. *Stupid*, as in *stupor*, connotes the end result of having been *stupified* into this state. *Strange* and *weird* represent progressive way-stations of emergence from projective identification.

Perhaps one of Dr. Paul's most "cutting-edge" concepts is his notion of fetal mental life. Derived from this concept as background, he explicates the idea of the prime importance of the inchoate sense organ *for pressure* and, emerging from that, the conception of the primitive emergence of the *superego* in the fetus. Pressure is one of the first sensory experience that the fetus feels; the other being sight. Pressure becomes activated during the birth process as a personified superego which menacingly clamps down on the fetus, challenging its willful escape, as it were, from the womb enclosure, and emergence into external life. This sense of an . . . inchoate "gatekeeper-challenge" reminds one of Bion's "Grid," especially the second vertical column, the "psi" (ψ) column, which represents the challenge given to the "definitory hypothesis" in vertical Column 1 of the Grid. What Paul is doing is, in part, innovatively applying Bion's concepts of the Grid and of fetal mental life and "putting flesh," so to speak, to the earliest conceivable dialectical relationship between subject and object, i.e., emerging fetus and squeezing maternal container. Thus, the fetus (and this is seen in retrospect) needs to claim its right to be born separate from, even though dependent upon, the needed object.

The readers of this work will certainly come to realize that its content is anything but prosaic. It belongs to the cutting-edge of psychoanalytic exploration and is unique in its oeuvre. Seldom does one find so many strands from such a variegated and gifted background coupled with an additional gift for innovative thinking and "imaginative conjecture" that speaks so credibly and immediately to the inner life of "every patient."

James S. Grotstein, MD

Acknowledgments

I feel deeply grateful to the late Wilfred R. Bion for helping me build mental equipment, without which, this work would not be possible. To say his role was inestimable is an understatement. I continue to work at the problems that he illuminated and realize that the means of observation of mental growth could only have been fostered by a kind attention which I had never experienced. Few individuals I have known had even a fraction of his generosity.

Seymour Friedman and James Grotstein have added immeasurably to my development, and to them I will always be grateful. I have had the luck to have both Ira Carson and James Grotstein as close friends and colleagues for many years. There has always been the spirit of discovery and enthusiasm for psychoanalytic theory and I can only feel enriched by their warmth and intellectual stimulation. Albert Mason has been a remarkable guide and mentor as well as a close friend. His supervision has been a continuing source of wisdom and has provided a model for the art of clinical practice.

Clara M. Szego instilled in me the discipline of scientific precision and the values associated with an experimental state of mind. It is rare to have the combination of idealism, discipline, and precision. She sought to pass these qualities down to her graduate students. Karl With, Rico Lebrun, and Hans Meyerhoff contributed enthusiasm, attention, and inspiration that are also inestimable. Joanne Grauer and Vitautis Paulekas aided in providing creative play and principles which I find add to psychoanalysis. Michael Metzger, Andra Akers, William Golant, and William Bronston have provided a continuing source of deep and creative friendship for many years.

My wife, Lyndell, has been a source of the deepest cooperation and has been my best editor. Clearly, without her continuing support, this work would not have been possible.

I would also like to express my sincere thanks to the following publications not only for permission to reprint the following papers but also for allowing me to publish them: Caesura Press and James S. Grotstein (Chapter 4), *Free Associations* (Chapter 8), *International Review of Psycho-Analysis* (Chapters 2 and 3), *Melanie Klein and Object Relations* (Chapters 5, 6, 7, and 8), *Esf* Publishers and the *Journal of Melanie Klein and Object Relations* (Chapters 9 and 10).

I offer special thanks to James S. Grotstein, who has kindly and generously accepted to write the Forward.

Before We Were Young

An Exploration of Primordial States of Mind

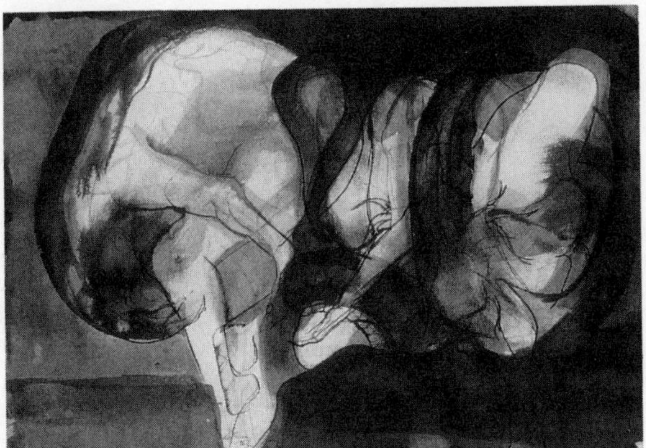

Chapter 1
Introduction

What has most engaged me about the practice of psychoanalysis has been the use of direct observation in the kind of detail that one usually has opportunity for only in relation to experience which is either impersonal or indirect. To have the privilege of direct observation in contact with another human being who is allowing exploration and cooperation is peculiar to the psychoanalytic process. Further, to undergo a procedure in which the opportunity for the kind of cooperation in a venture involving these two human beings in which the process can lead to psychic pain, often of very intense proportion, is highly unusual. Not only does the situation have similarities to surgery, but the analysand is like the assistant and the anesthesiologist. The operative procedure involves a kind of map-making which must depend on the establishment of mental coordinates. These coordinates may have generality from individual to individual but ultimately must involve the specific individual who is simply one of a kind. Scientific elaboration has become respectable for the most part, and even deified, as the agent of progress in the modern world. Respectability, however, is dependent upon repeatability and replicability. Since we operate with individuals (one of a kind), these criteria of replicability and repeatability have limited purchase, even though learned psychoanalysts often fail to remember something so simple and obvious. Our prejudice in favor of the individual must coordinate with a more general "sighting" orientation, a means of establishing the general terrain of mind which leads to the discovery of the individual, if we are respectful and fortunate enough.

We now have notions of a psychoanalyst being a scientist and surgeon, a person who must operate in the moment on what is observed. To complicate matters, the individual does not have a mental anatomy directly corresponding to what we understand in physical anatomy. The elaboration of these mental structures comprising both the defensive architecture and the qualities of mind which are individual require artistic abilities. An understanding of character has been well established by the history of those writers who have been successful in illuminating the truth about human beings in such a way that we are convinced that we have known an individual like *that* before but never quite. Often there is a relief from the loneliness that we all feel as well, when that writer succeeds in rendering the individual in so defined a manner that he/she is indelible. Other artistic means may attempt the same exploration from another vertex but have similar limitations when attempting to establish the individual. In that way, psychoanalysis must be an art insofar as its operative task is discovery and the elucidation of the individual.

W. R. Bion made it very clear that there could be no supervisor or psychoanalyst who could tell one what to say to a patient in psychoanalysis. He said that one had to find one's own cliches and forms of expression, a kind of establishment of improvisatory tools. These tools must be continuously forged and kept sharp if they are to be functional, and in fact are operative instruments. Bion's legacy informs us that prematurity of theory formation precludes observation and prevents the evolution of development of the material which leads the analyst to the elaboration of the individual. The tools we need, then, can never be formed because the facts which are needed to begin to understand the problems for which tools are needed can never emerge. This caution, that we respect what we do not and cannot know because it is not yet evolved or is unconscious, is essential. The analysand usually has no such inhibition. Therefore, the analyst's restraint is *essential* equipment necessary to the evolution of psychoanalytic phenomenology.

The precision of the phenomena described can open the terrain to mental operations both by analyst and analysand. The "interpretations" made are very different, depending on whether they arise from the archaic conscience or whether they originate from more civilized levels of mind. I mention this as the question is crucial to the psychoanalyst. From what sector of the mind does the thought or interpretation come, and as we learn from W. R. Bion's grid, what is it used for? Accuracy can have profound effects, even under the kindest and most truthful respect for the pain both individuals must suffer in psychoanalysis. As growth and development occur, it becomes very evident that we do not "understand" the means by which it occurs.

Verbal thought articulated in speech is a method of psychoanalytic interpretation. These words are received by the Pinna, auditory canal, tympanic membrane, ossicular chain, oval window, cochlea, cochlear nerves, medial Geniculate body, and auditory association cortex. This anatomic set of links transduces the sound vibrations to neuronal coded signals which reach specific areas of the brain. But how does the mind grow through verbal thought? Is it structural, as recent findings may show? If songbirds are placed together (of the same species yet who live on different islands), they will teach each other their songs. After learning these songs, they can be shown to have similar changes in dendritic arborization patterns in their auditory association cortices. Plasticity of the central nervous system is now being explored with powerful results (Kandel, 1991, 1995), and while we may postulate that plastic changes in neuronal structure may occur with learning, we must still account for the moment to moment observable changes that operate within the sphere of psychoanalytic observation. The profound power of our method is partially derived from millisecond to millisecond changes in thought and affect which are observable by our own psychoanalytic reception apparatus. Whether or not these changes are organized into biological structures or structure, as Hartmann suggested, is a matter for our consideration. It is to the precision of these "interpretations" that we may directly contribute observations about what "happens" upon their reception. These happenings must be observable within the limits of the psychoanalytic spectrum. If one can accurately detail the nature of the interactive effects of types of interpretation, we begin to have a body of data which can be discussed scientifically and on which different observers can compare their understanding.

The question "what do these interpretations do?" takes into consideration an action component. Something happens linked to the interpretive-reception process, both inter- and intra-psychically. We are thus psychoanalytic operators operating on a field of interactive mind which then is introjected by both analyst and analysand and has effect.

The reception apparatus of the analyst is partially unconscious. Analysand to analyst communication must then involve the linkage of unconscious to unconscious. In addition, there must be conscious elements which emerge for the translation to interpretation in the mind of both analyst and analysand. At the point which corresponds to what Freud described as preconscious, beginning elements evolve into a pattern which must be translated to verbal thought by the analyst. W. R. Bion (1970) has detailed the receptive process and described many of the difficulties in the translation of experience arising in the mind to verbal thought. I do not differentiate this, as both analyst and analysand must engage in this translation. I assume that the analyst's own analysis helps establish self-recognition; that is, the familiarity with his/her own receptor apparatus so that there can be greater sensitivity to material arising from the patient as distinct from the analyst's own mental process. The transference, then, is the experience passing between the analyst and analysand from second to second. Both are contributing to a mental field which is affected by the interactions which take place in it. Many species of experience are included; affects, sensations, thoughts, elaborated theories, dreams, hallucinations, and visions are only a part of that which contributes to the field.

I put these conditions forward in an abbreviated way to briefly describe the set within which psychoanalytic work is done. Specifically, these are many of the assumptions I have made in my own work which has made it possible to make the observations for further elaboration.

This book represents various approaches to observation and some version of what emerged as constantly conjoined. One of the most complex and interesting human acts is speech itself. W. R. Bion coined the phrase "verbal thought" to describe a distinction which is clinically observable. The process of translating pictorial to verbal thought, although known to Freud (1915), was emphasized by Bion in his clinical work, ("Language in the Schizophrenic" [1953], "Attacks on Linking" [1959], *Attention and Interpretation* [1970], and "Caesura" [1975]). The power of these contributions derives not only from accuracy but their nodal effect on clinical transformation. The point at which pictorial thought translates to verbal thought is a locus of a problem which is very significant—the difference, say, between thought and hallucination. One of the most basic ideas which can be clinically verified is the "simple" notion that translating experience to verbal thought intensifies affect, often to very painful degrees, which initiates attacks on linking (Bion, 1955). Part of Dr. Bion's legacy involves the practical approach to psychoanalytic transformations in verbal thought as they appear in symbol formation, leading to the elaboration of abstraction, but also more concrete forms as well.

In my view, part of W. R. Bion's wisdom involved the choice of nodal experiences to study. Phenomena, which can be seen to organize around specific points of observation, are detailed. A good scientist capitalizes on the nodal organizing observations that open up a whole domain of experience. Melanie Klein's notion of paranoid-schizoid to depressive position is an example of what I mean. Bion's focus on observation using PS as a defining state of mind is nonpathological when placed in the context of integration↔disintegration. It is a scientific tool. A theoretical construction may bring new facts into view. That point was very encouraging to me since the material to be explored is so vast as to be infinite. The field of exploration can profitably be shared by all who dare.

Language, verbal thought, and speech are crucial to the psychoanalytic venture. We think, we talk, and we sometimes remain silent. All are activities of both the analyst and analysand. Why not study the effect of language, the effect of the so-called prosodic elements of language; rhythm, intonation, verbal inflection, timbre?

The "Sense of Strangeness" (Chapter 2) came out of the words *stupid*, *dumb*, *weird*, and *strange* emerging as a pattern. The connections gradually shone through when began to realize that I did not know what the words meant and was shocked to discover the *Oxford English Dictionary*'s historical approach provided me with the tool that has led to an even greater mystery. Why should certain words retain a historical, archaic meaning when they are spoken, that corresponds to unconscious phantasy? The state of mind which is elaborated is very close to the original historical meaning of the word, although these words can be spoken by people without benefit of a philological education and hardly would have conscious awareness of the meaning. If this is so, then the question arises even more profoundly, what about the notion of the inheritance of acquired characteristics which was so roundly trounced by anti-Soviet American geneticists? It is true that if one cuts the tails off mice and they mate, the F_1 generation will indeed have tails. This does not explain, however, why the archaic meaning of a word is retained when, in fact, its use may have been discontinued in common parlance centuries ago. Those words *stupid*→*strange* comprise a series of referent indicators of the stage of emergence from a state of psychic fusion. This is a general observation that seems to cut across the specific differences between certain analysands and refers to states of mind which generally occur throughout development, despite the individual's native language.

In two chapters, "Intonational Elements of Communication in Psychoanalysis" (Chapter 8) and "On the Imitation of Human Speech" (Chapter 9), observations on the effects of tone and rhythm have been considered as a means of "setting a state of mind," by inducing specific affects which can operate by feedback loops to produce an organization which is stereotyped and has specific effects. Induced affect is different than an affect which arises in response to an experience coming into the mind from the outside. In response to an outside stimulus, there is greater flexibility in variation of affect without the stereotyping and is not utilized as a control mechanism. Induced affect has different qualities and is used as an organizer of experience. Frequently, induced affect can be used to block contact and set up a barrier which impedes communication. The use of an internal pharmacopoeia, specific organized fantasies, to perform actions affecting either the analyst or analysand have great variety depending on the individual. Listening to analytic material with a musical ear is explored briefly and forms a serious question for the training and education of psychoanalysts. Do we benefit from musical education to increase our sensitivity to the interactive patterns of sound which are more precisely described by musical notation and by musicians than any other field? How do you learn to listen and to what? This approach might be profitably considered as an important adjunct to the field.

An extension of the notion of language as a form of action that Bion (1955) referred to in "Language and the Schizophrenic" led to the theory that language has specific drug-like effects which can be organized into a virtual phantasy which utilizes induced affect to produce a constancy of mental organization defensively. An autistic protection against interactive incursion leads to imitation of communication so that an individual's mental location cannot be determined. A conversation appears to have meaning but does not. Rather, sensations are produced, only giving the illusion of an interactive process. There is a simulation and technique established for the "appearance" of communication.

The primal scene has long been an important feature of psychoanalytic theory (Freud, S., 1918). The elements of sense based on W. R. Bion's theory of "common sense" (1962) organize experience in a particular way. When referring to dimensionalization, there is a shift from deadness, flatness, and lifelessness to vibrancy, depth, and three-dimensionality. In our discussions, Dr. Carson and I noted dedimensionalization associated with more complete geographic, projective identification (the phantasy of being totally inside an object and indistinguishable from it). Phantasies of intercourse (not necessarily genital) are coded by reference to a predominant sense mode. The linkage between the parents in phantasy is represented by specific sense modes coming together in patterns which have a profound effect on the thinking process. There is an assemblage of the parental intercourse using specific senses as representatives. Blocking contact between the mother and the father and their representative senses blockades the thinking process as it arises in the moment during the session. The organization of thought utilizing those specific senses may well be curtailed. For example, vision and audition may be prevented from connecting.

Throughout this book, there is a consistent concern about the establishment of mental contact between analyst and analysand as a primary organizer of developmental flow both in the session and as a necessary condition for growth. We found that specific senses are identified as a reference to the experience of the primary object. Vision and hearing are long range senses while touch and taste are short range. Olfaction tends to be used at mid-range. The utilization of a long-range sense at short range can produce a failure to connect as well as the misuse of a short-range sense at long range. It is possible to observe how the maternal and paternal objects are assembled by their sense representatives and can be studied according to their use. The thinking processes which evolve reflect this linkage and are influenced by the nature of the organization of senses, especially with regard to specific accuracy. The means of establishing contact by analysis of the organization of the connection between the senses is an example of the kind of specific mental operation which can make a fundamental difference.

A major theme presented in this book elaborates prenatal influences as they appear in the mental process of the adult. It is only in the last 20 years that the field of prenatal influences has been revivified in psychoanalysis. When Bion presented work on this theme as imaginative conjecture and a kind of "science fiction," there was considerable violence evoked in audiences who tended to feel assaulted and responded in kind. I was amazed and horrified at the rage and disrespect which greeted these ideas, and yet even now there can be just as powerful a reaction. I have been less uncertain as to the source of this violence when, after having worked as long with the experience, the fundamental nature of the work has become even more evident.

J. S. Grotstein edited what was to be a festschrift for W. R. Bion which sadly turned out to be a memorial volume. "A Mental Atlas of the Process of Psychological Birth" (Chapter 4) was published as an attempt to come to some understanding of the basic elements of prenatal phantasy, especially with regard to prelabor and the actual "traumatic" elements of labor itself.

The notion that seems so simple in retrospect, so much so that its symmetry can seem syllogistic, is that there are vestiges of primitive embryologic structures such as notochordomas and Branchial cleft cysts in the adult human being which express themselves in adult life as pathological forms. There can also be psychical states which are remnants or vestiges of the fetal state of mind or elements of the maternal environment laid down as mnemic residues which have varying degrees of expressivity. In certain situations, the observations and understanding to which Piontelli has greatly added in her book *Backwards in Time* and in her articles (1987, 1988), these stages of mental development can dominate the mind of an adult, and these memories and possibly "interpretations" arrived at by the fetal mind can be expressed. These states of mind have been described previously by Bion, Grotstein, Meisels, Piontelli, and myself, so far without a detailed clear understanding of why these primordial experiences are so evident in selected cases. We have a beginning notion of the regulation of these states and a somewhat greater awareness of the nature of the phenomena which are evidenced in psychoanalytic circumstances. Bion (1975) hinted at maternal-fetal forms of projective identification. A natural field of study is the psychoanalysis of pregnancy. I have had the good fortune of analyzing four women before, during, and through their pregnancies, and it is clear that maternal fantasy directly plays on the fetal activity. Two examples come to mind.

One, a woman in her middle thirties, experienced the fetus as damaging her, about which she felt extreme anxiety. Her feeling that the fetus was parasitically draining her of life made her hate her pregnancy, and she observed a marked increase of this hatred with quickening. As the fetus grew and she felt its movements, she was seized by hatred and was able to observe with fear and regret that the fetal movement decreased and stopped during her bouts of hatred. Analysis of her primitive infantile oral phantasies of draining and destroying her mother's body relieved her anxiety, and the fetus was observed to resume normal movement.

The second patient, during the seventh month of pregnancy, played a game with the fetus during which she noticed that when she shifted to pictorial from nonpictorial thought (she could do this at will), the fetus began active movements which were timed on and off directly with changing her mental process from visual to nonvisual and vice versa. The baby would kick when she "turned on" visual thought and stopped when she stopped. The patient took delight in "showing" me this game which aroused in her a sense of pleasure and awe.

A preview list of phenomena associated with prenatal experience is briefly presented as a guide to introduce the reader to the topic.

1. The experience of pressure.
2. Pressured lifestyle.
3. A sense of infinite vs. finite time.
4. The sense of dread.
5. The sense of strangeness.
6. Either/or versus *and* thinking.
7. Fear of mutilation.
   a. Psychosomatic expressions of muscular dystonia.
8. Dread associated with psychic movement.
9. Agoraphobia.

10. The phenotype of greed.
11. A sense or foreknowledge or a sense of prescience and its effect on decision making.
12. The moralization of phenomenology.
13. Inability to make a selection based on desire.
14. Anhedonia and the driven lifestyle.
15. Beating fantasies and elements of sadomasochism.
16. Voluptuousness and character traits as Piontelli has demonstrated ultrasonographically.
17. Obsessional thought as a means of stopping psychic movement and as a process by which the rhythmic elements of labor contractions and delivery are evidenced expressed in "verbal banging."
18. Mental turbulence.
19. A penitential life representing elements of formation of the primordial superego.

I certainly think that while this rather limited list of experiences and phenomena can be related to a level of mind which has its origins in prenatal life, I do not mean to suggest that postnatal experiences do not have vast importance. Rather, I would say that the postnatal experiences are nourished by or activated by the presence of phenomena at the fetal level of mind.

There appears to be a difference between early, middle, and late prenatal epochs and those phenomena associated with the onset and experience of labor. To classify these phenomena definitively at this time I think is a bit premature, although the elements associated with the activation of labor and the birth process are the most impressive and some of the clearest.

We are all familiar with individuals who live with the expectation of having no pain or stress and feel that everything should be done for them. There should be no gaps between expectation and fulfillment. Even fulfillment is a problem since there never should have been need to require fulfillment. There is no concept of development of capacities or any form of process which involves incremental change. Any form of change is hated and evokes dread and terror. In extreme situations, one finds them isolating themselves with the blinds drawn, shut up in their rooms, refusing contact. Eating and breathing are often very conflictual, and there are frequent references in dreams to underwater life, very often associated with phylogenetically primitive biological forms. Any form of boundary is hated and references to linear time are denied. The expectation "as it was in the beginning, so shall it be forever" holds true. There is the operation of phantasied infinite time. These problems begin to occur when there is the reality of the demands of the external world brought to them. At that intersection, we find the evolution of defensive structures meant to keep the analysand hermetically sealed. When this seal is broken, the individual makes "interpretations" arising from very early sources and experiences life as punishment and cruelty being inflicted upon them.

In "Primordial Development of the Penitential Transference" (Chapter 5) it occurred to me that the Archaic Superego that Melanie Klein elaborated had its origins in prenatal life. The Talion code demands an eye for an eye and a tooth for a tooth. There is some concept of fairness in revenge. The punishment seems to be a systematic form of revenge in that code which was considered a considerable advance over the Draconian code in which the punishment for all crimes was death. The interpretations coming from the primordial superego have psychic movement and change as a trigger. All references to change are interpreted as leading straight to death and instigate the "interpretations" which are meant to stop all movement. This is felt as a "protection" and all incursion by the analytic process is felt as a threat to life itself. The individual seeks to reestablish the prenatal orientation and interprets his/her adult self as a fabrication or lie. The result is lifelong depression and a failure to acknowledge features of his adult life.

I wish to reference the totalitarian nature of the maintenance of the inside womb state as the narcissistic, perfectionistic ideal of ever-lasting life without change, as being linked to the presence of a strict either-or logic which cannot allow the possibility of "and."

The "and" additive logic would lead to infinite change and growth and is the deadly enemy of the maximum security system seen both as a prison and as a safe haven. The question as to the differentiation between elements of the personality and more stereotyped elements which become defenses in the context of group institutional forms becomes highly relevant here. Not only the question of when is the character or personality born, but how do we differentiate the indelible impress of derivatives of the birth experience stamped on the fragile emerging personality. I am making a primary distinction between personality and the elements of superego which I believe to be distinct.

Countless times, W. R. Bion, in personal communications as well as in public, emphasized the need for the analyst to develop an understanding of a mental coordinate system. These chapters all involve that attempt to establish a clinical set of coordinates that are relevant to the interpretation of clinical phenomena. In that sense, the establishment of coordinates, even on a temporary, hypothetical basis, is an important aspect of instrument-building. How does one date the superego? Is it Talionic or Draconian? Is there a sophisticated judgment involved? Do we find the individual operating on infinite time or, as J. S. Grotstein jokes, on "infant standard time"? Are there dominant senses involved in the organization of phantasy? Do individuals have the capacity for multiple tracking in which practiced non-pathological splitting is utilized, or do they have a one-track mind? What happens when a decision needs to be made? Do they break off contact as though something dreadful would occur or can they think and act subsequently on what they have decided? We are accustomed to considering the uncertainty which is a necessary condition of all decisions. That uncertainty alone does not explain the intensity of the level of dread and fear of death that results. The questions referred to help in locating the time zone of the assumptions of the analysand and may aid in the indication of mental location.

A further elaboration of the prenatal vestiges of experience emerging into adult life can be found in Chapter 6 on "Studies on the Phenomenology of Mental Pressure." The experience of mental pressure in adult life today has been the subject of political and social debate. The increasing density of information flooding in with inadequate means of selection is a common social ill. The demands of life today seem to exclude nonpressured experience and there are frequent complaints of being harried. It is beyond the scope of this book to delve into the "social experiences" to which I refer, yet I think it may be useful to consider the contribution of the prenatal vestiges of pressure and the nonsensuous transduction of experience to the sensation of pressure. I think there may be a resonance between these external aspects of pressure and the internal sources which are discussed here.

We all make a constant flux of interpretations of the data we receive through our senses. There is a need to determine the effect of these interpretations so that their accuracy can be ascertained. In addition, many unconscious interpretations arise from sources which may have a background of sense data.

In Chapter 7 on "Practical Psychoanalytic Epistemology," an effort is made to distinguish sources of mental experience in order to determine whether we are dealing with fact, opinion, or interpretation. I am most concerned about how to distinguish between experience which is induced —that is, "manufactured"—to produce a desired result and actual incoming experience which must be accurately interpreted to lead to appropriate thinking and action. A major theme considered in Chapter 7 extends to the problems of defining virtual fantasies/phantasies in order to make a distinction between actual real time experience and simulation. This distinction is of crucial significance since sensations and affective states can be induced by autostimulation. The affect is powerful and indistinguishable from an object related experience. This distinction can make it possible to sort both internal and external propaganda leading to far greater freedom of thought and action.

The influence of mass media and the dawn of the information age puts at risk some fundamental elements of mental development such as the primary distinction between the awareness of the difference between presence and absence. While this is not new, the deluge of available substitutes for contact through television, film, radio, and the Internet can be daunting. Properly used, each of these media can be a great development in the education and entertainment of human beings. Like language, the potential for misuse is just as great. The profusion of psychoanalytic material derived from these sources is impressive. Note the crowds of people interviewed on television about their witness to events taking on the imitative qualities of the television journalists so that it becomes difficult to determine whether the interviewee is a bystander or a professional journalist. One cannot avoid influence even if it were desirable, and there is a concern that influence leads to imitation which is a natural part of the learning process. When this imitation becomes "the" way of life and the propaganda cannot be distinguished from the truth, we lose our freedom. I do not consider these distinctions academic. I think these questions are of major importance in the study of human beings.

This volume represents a collection of psychoanalytic work engaged in over the last 25 years. Most of the work is clinical although the earliest paper, "Transformational Aspects of Phantasy in Relation to Dyadic Communication Under the Influence of Marijuana" (Chapter 10), was part of a study conducted in the UCLA Department of Psychiatry during 1970-1973. I had the good fortune to have the collaboration of Ira M. Carson and W.R. Bion to help in the development of a methodology for the analysis of phantasy in two-person groups. These groups were videotaped while they were under the influence of marijuana. We were searching for invariants that would be evident and might serve as a research tool for investigating other invariants in groups in which either physical substances or analogous processes to physical substances could be studied. The beginning results are presented here as a kind of milestone for the use of a field theory involving the use of interactive phantasy. This work had a profound influence on my development as a psychoanalyst and is presented here in brief. The remainder of the chapters presented are derived entirely from clinical articles.

Chapter 2
The Sense of Strangeness

In this chapter we hope to elucidate the relationship between certain ordinary words that have come up in the treatment of a variety of our patients. The words in question are: *stupid*, *dumb*, *weird*, and *strange*. We have observed that there is a constantly conjoined relationship between these words which extends throughout a therapeutic session, even throughout years of an analytic process, and cuts across the differences between the individual analyses of patients, all of whom have in common the diagnoses of borderline psychotic or ambulatory schizophrenics. These words may be considered to represent a mental process describing the change in the use of the perceptual apparatus with respect to different stages of emergence from states of projective identification (psychic fusion).

Early in the analyses of three patients there has been pronounced exaggerated material at the beginning of the sessions with reference to the word *dumb* and/or *stupid*. The usage of terms such as *dumb* or *stupid* levied with great vociferousness has the flavor of self judgement and violent self attack, which has been later transformed in different stages of the analyses to the word *dumb* or "I have nothing to say." Initially we thought this was primarily an attempt to maintain out of awareness the elements that were emerging into consciousness at that time. This experience occurs most frequently at the beginning of the session. Taking the word *dumb* as a primitive pun and applying it to the concept of obscuring material, the word may alert the therapist to the recognition of a form of obscuration in the session.

Our first example is Miss A., a 40-year-old spinster school teacher, who has been in treatment for two years and had become progressively isolated. She was unable to work and unable to leave her rooms. She was out of contact with every member of her family and lived in a reportedly disheveled apartment, her only friends were books that she did not read and she was preoccupied with a series of paranoid persecutory delusions. She felt that everyone she knew hated her violently and wished her dead. A session after two years of treatment demonstrates the use of the words in question:

> [She begins:] I have nothing to say [Long pause]. I had a dream Friday night that *I was on top of a mountain and going down very quickly in a train . . . I prayed and wished to stop, but the train would not stop . . . I felt terror and pushed a green button in a box at my immediate side. The question was, would we be able to go on? The train came to a terrific stop, and a group of people that I was with and I got out and we walked past the train. We had stopped inside a tunnel, we could see daylight within, the tunnel was brightly lit and had water running through it . . . I was amazed at what I saw. As I walked beyond the train, I noted that there was a distance that lay ahead in which there were no tracks and many rocks, but we still decided to go on . . . from the other end, the train looked like a bed . . . I was preoccupied in the train with hair styles and putting on ear-rings. I decided to go on anyway.*

She associated hearing to ear-rings and then identified herself with her students who are now able to hear. Her references were clear in this hour and in the previous several weeks, to a change which indicated that her classes had been responding very favorably to her teaching capacities. Previously she had been preoccupied with fears of losing her job and felt that her students were not learning and hated her for being a poor teacher.

> It's weird, nothing makes sense any longer, I can't understand the world any longer, everything seems topsy-turvy . . . I was thinking about whether or not it seems like I am in a new world . . . I have been parking my car in a different place . . . I had an image of walking from my car . . . I have been having a problem with one child in the class . . . last year, Mrs. White [her therapist], I felt it was terrible that an ultraconservative woman, who went a great length to stop sex on the campus . . . Wendy is my student who I talk to and then I finally realized that I could work with her and that she might not be such a bad counselor after all. Last year she was punishing, this year she is not, but that in a way I can recognize in myself a less "either/or" type of attitude toward her. I am never quite sure where things are at that school, I always go through feelings of being scared to death that I am being observed and criticized. For when I started teaching, I have had a tremendously horrible sense of time . . . it doesn't make me nearly so anxious as before, there is only so much that I can do in a day and I can't help it that I can't do everything. I was also thinking that it's Wednesday

and I look forward to coming in here, I felt that's silly . . . in a very short while you won't be here I will have left, in fact in about two minutes I will, that's strange.

Looking more closely at the material in this session we note that it begins with an opening statement followed by a dream with associations relating to her increased ability to use her auditory sense and subsequent improved functioning. She continues with the statement "It's weird . . . ," referring to the change in her perception of the world including a notation of the difference between the present and the past, her anxiety about the unfamiliarity with her new perceptual tools and the dismay over the acknowledgment of the distinction between my presence and absence. She denotes with the word *strange* the awareness of impending separation as if to say that previously she never would have thought it possible.

In the dream we note representation of the failure of her wish to stop a process through prayer and her terror in terms of her experience of helplessness to stop the train. In the dream, the train stood for the treatment which she wished to control through alternating violent stops and starts. The uncertainty of the future is represented by the absence of tracks and anticipated difficulties by rough terrain. There are several references denoted by the presence of bed-analysis and also by her involvement with ear-rings.

This state of unfamiliarity and uncertainty represented by the dream as part of the past is continued in the present consciously in the session, in a definite shift in a state of mind, introduced by: "It's weird, nothing makes sense . . . ." Here the patient spoke with a sense of bewildered sadness about how her life was changing vis-à-vis her perception of the therapy, the therapist (Mrs. White), her increasing tolerance of uncertainty and the beginning of an improved sense of time. Her reference to separation is denoted by the word *strange*, which also was uttered with a sense of accepting puzzlement. Earlier in the treatment opening statements very often contained a strong peppering of the word *stupid* or *dumb* used as epithets to attack her inability to conform to her massive expectations of herself.

These statements *stupid*, *dumb*, *weird*, and *strange* represent signposts with respect to the relative degree of projective identification in this particular patient. In a progressive transformation throughout the hour we began with *dumb*, which is substituted for the vicious attacks made on herself previously and which are now visible as having obscured omnipotent mechanisms noted in the dream.

According to *Webster's New World Dictionary of the American Language* (1968), *dumb* means reticent silence, misty, dark, obscured, lacking the power of speech, unwilling to talk, silent, reticent, not accompanied by speech, temporarily speechless as from fear, grief, etc. and/or producing no sound; *stupid* means to be stunned or amazed in a state of stupor, dazed, stunned, stupefied; *strange,* in its original middle English definition states "that which is without, extra, on the outside, foreign, alien, not previously known, seen, heard, experienced or unfamiliar"; *weird* comes from the middle English again in its most primitive definition and has to do with the future tense from the German *werden* or the old English *wyrd*, which has to do with that which is about to occur, that which is prophesied, uncanny, but also refers to foggy, misty and definitely seems to represent a distinct distant state of mind.

Here we have words which seem to be used in their original middle English definitions, in their most primitive forms, which are references to states of mind that are changing from the inside to the outside; *dumb* representing the maximal inside state of mind (relatively complete geographical confusion, Meltzer, 1967). *Weird* is a premonitory word in this particular context and thus seems to represent the apperception of a state of mind which has to do with the unfolding of a process that might be described as emergence from a mental state of psychic fusion or projective identification.

Freud (1908) has drawn attention to the shift in the meaning of the word from its contemporary context to a more archaic usage:

> Thus in following the usage of language, neurosis, here as elsewhere, is taking words in their original, significant sense, and where it appears to be using a word figuratively it is usually simply restoring its old meaning (p. 174).
>
> . . . the course of linguistic evolution has made things very easy for dreams. For language has a whole number of words at its command which originally had a pictorial or concrete significance, but are used to-day in a colorless and abstract sense. All that the dream need do is give these words their former, full meaning or to go back a little way to an earlier phase in their development (Freud, 1900, p. 407).

We should like to put forward another example of the sense of strangeness as a reference to the more primitive meaning of the word *strange* referring to outside.

Mr. D, a 35-year-old corporate executive, has been in intensive treatment for a period of two years. He had been excessively dependent upon a woman ten years older than himself who had left him, which precipitated a serious (100 Tuinal) suicidal attempt. He also had been seen in psychotherapy five years previously. The patient had lived his entire life in conformity with the expectations of other people and had attempted to maintain a perfect conformation to the "shape of another person's style of life," the expectations of an employer, a woman, or with anyone with whom he had a relation. In short, the patient has lived most of his life in a very powerful form of virtually complete projective identification in which he existed in phantasy, primarily "inside" his objects. Accordingly, a previous marriage that the patient had was a failure after a month. He had no contact with his family for several years. His life was impoverished with respect to friends and working associates, and he had failed in most of his previous work because of his great incapacity to deal with others. I should like to present part of a Friday weekend session.

> I don't know what to say; I have nothing to say. [Pause.] I had a dream in which *my company, X, owned two other companies, E and I, and they were going to send me off to them. They were in other cities and I did not want to go. They wanted me to transfer there.* In reality, however, the parent company did not own these companies, although they had sent me out previously to negotiate to see whether we ought to buy them. Shipping me off and not wanting to go is understandable, but it seemed like a *strange* thing to realize, I'm being shipped off the weekend.

I interpreted, "The company, X, is experienced as if they are in possession of you and they can do with you what they wish. They are experienced as the treatment is today," with reference to the weekend break.

> "Yes, I'm being shipped off for the weekend," he said, "but I don't want to go, so I won't. This morning I thought, wouldn't it be fun to ranch in Colorado. Last night I went out with a girl, S., whose father is a rancher in Texas."

This is a clear example of projective identification in which the patient is located in phantasy inside this girl, S., to avoid the experience of the separation from the treatment over the weekend. One could continue the analysis of this very rich material extensively. However, at the time the patient used the word *strange*, I inquired about the patient's usage of this word and nothing occurred to him that was peculiar about the dream, even though he used the words. What seemed peculiar was that the parent company, X, did not own those companies. So here again, *strange* shines out as a reference point to a position in mental space referring to being outside a container. This is a reference in the dream to separation in phantasy from the parent, which the weekend break stimulated. The parent company stands for a representation of the ultimate parent who contained the patient totally. His rebellion and "refusal" to leave for the weekend is an indication of his enormous anxiety about separation, which is only mitigated by the complete replacement of the analytic situation with a dating arrangement which is equated with the treatment.

There exists a change in the state of mind along a coordinate denoted by the words *amazing* and *stupid*. The word *stupid* has a series of definitions, the most primitive of which has to do with a stuporous state, but later historical usages include *dazed* and *amazed* as indications of states of mind. Thus contained in a word such as *stupid* there may be important clues as to changes of state of mind as the usage of the word changes through time. The word *stupid*, used virtually as an epithet interspersed through a session and notable especially within the beginning few moments, was originally taken to refer to a harsh, judgmental, self-attacking aspect of the personality. The word *stupid* seemed to refer to situations in which the patient had unreasonably high expectations of his mental capacities, especially referent to the capacity to predict the future. Thus *stupid* referred to instances in which a kind of "mistake" was perceived (by the patient) and a gap existed between what occurred and what the patient expected to occur. Further, the word *stupid*, akin to the usage of the word *dumb* as referred to above, may designate the presence of a mode of obscuration in which a train of thought is being hidden relative to the presentation of the conscious aspects of phantasy. The word *stupid* has to do then, with a state of mind related to a stupor, although the patient may not seem to be dulled, deadened or blunted. Associated with stupor, signified by the presence of the word *stupid* exist states of mental confusion between self and other (which may be included in the more broadly defined concept of projective identification). The term "projective identification" has been used primarily by proponents of Kleinian psychoanalytic theory to describe a vast variety of forms of confusional interchanges between self and object. Although Melanie Klein (1957) and Meltzer (1967) have described a categorization of the types of this phenomenon, I feel there is an opportunity to further distinguish several stages of mental confusion moving along a continuum of self inside object (in phantasy) to self outside object.

A patient (Mr. D) mentioned above illustrated this *stupid-amazing* transformation over a series of sessions in which it was clear that he was emerging out of a state of stupor in which he had very little contact with "feelings," into a state in which he had far greater contact with his perceptual abilities and feelings. The patient had represented a Home Owners' Association that was in the process of fighting an encroaching housing development, which was experienced by the Association as spoiling the beauty of the area. "I hate smoke screens like those the lawyers put up." There were numerous references to stupidity as the patient was describing the machinations of the Housing Development Advisory Committee, the legal loopholes involved and the political intervention involving graft in city government. I believed him to be using the word *stupidity* in this particular context as having the meaning of another person or another agency being asleep to his needs and as a result producing suffering in the end. The patient's feelings were reported by him to be deadened at the meeting at the time when these issues were raised, as indeed they were in the session as the patient was re-experiencing the situation in the transference. The patient then reported, giving an impassioned account of the needs of the members of the Housing Association with whom he was identified. As he did so, he noted a variety of feelings in the audience, as indeed there were during his report of the account in the session, including fear, sadness and his own *amazement* at the state of emotion palpable in the audience. Amazement, then, for the patient was a signifier of his state of stupor. He punctuated his account of this phase of the experience with the word *amazing*. He noted that for the first time he was able to link his thoughts and feelings in a public situation. It was clearly observable to me that during the session the same phenomena were occurring.

The *amazing-stupid* axis, as it were, may be an example of representing a coordinate of mental confusion, with *amazing* being the designator of a state of mind in which there is a gap between the self and the object, and *stupid* designating a mental state in which there exists a confusional state in which there is no space between the self and the object.

With references to stupidity, sleep and stupor it seems evident that there exists a state of confusion in the mind of the patient which includes a misunderstanding of that which takes place between two objects. This "mis-understanding" conforms to the description of rather complete projective identification and involves confusion of the "outside" with the "inside." Stupidity seems to be an active state of not knowing. Stupidity may subserve a mental state which includes ingredients of that which is not to be known (future), oscillating with that which has taken place and is actively kept from awareness. A process of obscuration is noted to occur but one does not know what has taken place which is being obscured.

Do we say we are *dumb* when we have no awareness of the object in identifiable sensory modes such as vision, hearing, etc.? Further, it seems that *stupid* represents the burgeoning awareness of the presence of an object that has not yet emerged into the domain of the sensory apparatus in phantasy. This partial awareness, then, represents a further state of the evolution of "knowledge" of an object as it passes into view of the perceptual apparatus but has not yet been located in space or time. *Weird* may be designating a border state between the inside and outside, indicating the capacity for moving bidirectionally between the two psychic *loci.*

The transformation of *weird* into *strange* seems to be linked with a process which involves the coalescing of a whole object from the experience of part objects and the bringing together of a psychic split which is facilitated by keeping the sense data received through one perceptual organ separate from the data received through another. Thus if one knows an object through both hearing and vision, the part object state would involve the maintenance of a lack of integration of the data from these two senses at a minimum, and the transformation to the whole object state then involves the integration of both vision and hearing which coheres the sense representation of the object. The designating word *strange* is noted after the mental object has coalesced and there has been recognition of the split. *Weird* represents the inability to formulate a whole object because of insufficient sensory coordination from a minimum of two sense representatives. Further, *weird* represents a state of mind which begins by the introduction of an additional sense representation where the "data" have not yet been integrated for use. Thus this represents a state of evolution of mental experience from the point of view of a single sense representation (visual) to the admixture of a second sense representation (auditory). We are postulating that the state of mind represented by the word *weird* may signal the beginning of intuition.

Strange represents a more concrete separation from the object with the awareness of emergence into a state of unfamiliarity. If a particular experience of an emerging mental object obtrudes as *weirdness* to a mental state which is set, as it were, at a "baseline" which includes a specific type of linking between the sensory representatives in phantasy, then that which is designated as *weird* is being perceived as being in a state of motion. Further, that which is considered *weird* has then already obtruded beyond the boundary which is experienced as known. If we refer to different states of mind we can use the analogy of a microscope as Freud (1900) has done.

Depending upon the setting of the aperture, the objective lens and the amount of light exposure, we may note different depths or layers included in the field and therefore a different phenomenology. What is *weird* for one state of mind is not necessarily *weird* for another. If there is a representation of a change in the position and integration of a mental object approaching the border to a different psychic locale, this burgeoning sense of internal psychic movement in phantasy may trigger anxiety. This process locates change and betrays the presence of a mental object which one may not wish to know, which may further activate the "focusing" process.

The concept of *weirdness* as has been previously described involved a change in the perception of time. Coincident with the process of awareness, something exists in consciousness which did not previously exist. Therefore, a comparison between the state of something being present in awareness and something being absent from awareness is inherently contained in this issue. Is there the equivalent of a state of mental movement from mental location to mental location which includes by necessity the introduction of a quantity of time into consciousness? What senses do we need to "know" time? If the unconscious has no time sense and the emergence of an emotional experience into consciousness introduces time, how then is this brought about? It seems likely that at least two sense modalities are required in order to "know" time in that there is the use of an inherent comparison between vision and hearing or touch and hearing. These senses must be able to probe space in order to produce some kind of mental location on a coordinate system that is mentally represented by a means which is still unknown.

Consciousness involves this "binocularity," to use a term which Bion (1962) has introduced, of at least two senses brought together in relation to time through mental space.

These words, *stupid*, *dumb*, *weird* and *strange*, are referring to a mental process involving a fluctuating series of links between sense representations converging, integrating and diverging. In the process of the emergence of a mental object into consciousness, the pattern of sensory integration is altered by the introduction of the "new" experience. Then *weirdness* or *strangeness* are markers which denote a change in the relationships between the sensory systems represented through phantasy.

Chapter 3

A Contribution to the Study of Dimension

Freud (1915), in his supplement to his metapsychological paper on the unconscious, considers the process by which information is retrieved from the system UCS by means of its attachment to a word presentation and thereby links to the visual apparatus in phantasy (p. 209). The idea of the word and the visual idea are connected as an experience becomes conscious. He makes the point that the visual channel is the dominant aperture through which sensory information must pass before it can achieve connexion with the representatives of other sense modalities.

Bion (personal communication, 1973) has drawn attention to the dominance of the visual apparatus in relation to other senses, doing so in the context of studies on the transformation of the thinking process. In his formulation of the grid (Bion, 1963), he has indicated that beyond a certain point, that is, "c" elements, thinking must go on in a nonvisual matrix. That is, the thinking process is no longer represented in visual terms when the level of abstraction reaches the stage of conception leading to concept formation. For example, what is being written here is not presented in visual language but if one were to say, "the sun set with cloudy amber glow as it slid into the water through the fog," visualization would be possible. In this way we have utilized a form of language which is capable of leading to visual representation in the mind and have noted the transformation to another kind of language which in fact does not generally lead to visualization. In this way we have a point of reference from which the shift from visible to invisible becomes evident. We wish to explore here the means by which the connexion of thought elements contained in the visual channel are mated with other sensory modalities in the process of the development of dimensionalization of experience. When referring to dimensionalization, we mean the change from a quality of deadness, flatness, and colorlessness (which has been associated with the state of being inside an object in phantasy) to an experience of liveliness, three dimensional form, depth and a sense of meaning. For this change to occur more than one sense must come together in phantasy thereby adding a quality of experience and forming a connexion based on the linkage between the experiences connected by means of the different sensory representations. The dimensionalization of experience is a concept which has previously been explored by Bion (1962), Meltzer (1975), Paul and Carson (1976; see Chapter 2) and Grotstein (1977).

We will posit the hypothesis that certain forms of experience with special reference to phantasies of intercourse between the parents are coded in specific sense modalities as defined for each patient. We will attempt to extend the theory that the parental intercourse is a model for the instigation of the thinking process (Bion, 1962) by linking each specific parent to a separate sense modality. We do not mean that one sense modality is exclusively related to one parent. We are noting the presence of a preponderance of a primary sense modality as related to the patient's experience of the parent in phantasy. Further, when we speak in this presentation of sense modalities in the patient, we are referring to the manner by which the objects in the external world are represented in phantasy as transformed by the mental apparatus of the subject in question and reported in the context of a psychoanalytic session.

In certain borderline and psychotic patients there is a process in which information coming into auditory channels is immediately transformed from auditory information to visual information and then experienced in visual terms as if it were expelled out through the eye (in phantasy). The patient will behave as if he were dealing with solid material which could actually be expelled in the form of an hallucination. This mechanism is exceedingly subtle and is denoted by several qualities which, in their exaggerated form, can be seen as muscular activity. In one patient, a profound muscular expelling movement, a rapid, forceful, thrusting, and jactating movement of the head and upper body seem to correlate with the phantasy of the expulsion of such a mental object through the eye and into a corner of the room in a manner similar to that previously described by Bion (1967) in his paper "On hallucination."

There are, however, very subtle forms of this particular difficulty which are extremely insidious and show themselves to be present and associated with "as if" communication which is a variant of insincerity out of the awareness of the patient. A quality associated with "as if" communication involves a sense that no meaning has transpired in the emotional situation which has occurred in the analysis. No contact in terms of actual affective experience is made. This kind of distant communication is frequently associated with the splitting we were describing and is mentioned as a constant observation although it is not the main subject of this chapter. Reference is made to "as if" communication at this time because of the constant association between the splitting of sense modalities and the presence of "as if" communication. Although this will be the subject of a later study, a simple definition would include the patient's not saying what he means and/or not meaning what he says. One or the other of these particular categories of insincerity must be present in order for "as if" communication to be present. The conversation is often noted to be put in the subjunctive or, the patient may be talking as if only one person was present in the room. Here we are attempting to make a link with Bion's (1962) theory of "common sense" that the utilization of information from one sense must be correlated with information integrated from another sense in order to produce the experience of dimension or the sense of "reality" of an experience.

What is the evidence that had led us to hypothesize that vision can represent one object (i.e. the father and hearing), or another sense may represent another object (i.e. the mother). Clinically, this is reflected when an object is represented by a marked preponderance of a single sense. For example, patient A always refers to father in terms of yelling, screaming, or not speaking at all for days at a time. In addition, father was represented as not hearing or listening to what the patient had to say. This aspect of relatedness of patient to the father involved representative mediation through sound as the preponderant modality. By contrast, mother was represented in visual terms—she sees me, I see her, she gives me dirty looks, she smiles at me, she gets tears in her eyes, etc. It was noted that father was rarely represented in visual terms. In dreams, if mother and father appeared together, mother would be smiling or frowning whereas father was represented as speaking. For example, the patient dreamed she was driving up to her parents' home. Mother came out of the door behind father, smiling, and father could not stop talking. The patient remembered feeling rage in the dream "why can't mother say something?" She was unable to amplify the experience that she could never develop the added dimension of experience in speech with mother as she had with father. She felt a substantial emotional contact with father which was absent with mother. She also noted that mother in real life did speak as often as father but the emotional contact through verbal exchange was felt to be thin and without meaning. Her primary connection to mother, therefore, was mainly visual while primary contact with father was auditory. Though there may be many other explanations, this distinction was noted to be in operation from the earliest contact in analysis. Mother was reported to have said to the patient at the age of five: "You only listen to father and not to me."

We have observed that when vision as the mother sense and audition as the father sense are able to be connected, or mated, then the means exist for the thinking process to evolve within the context of the session. In the assemblage of the parental intercourse between the senses as representations, we note the activation of the thinking process. The attempt to interrupt the links between the senses as representations of the links between the parents, e.g. between audition which may stand for one parent, and vision, standing for the other, may be a way of keeping a relationship between the parents from occurring in phantasy.

In clinical observation, we note the predominance of one sense representing a parent in a word set which conveys a quality of sense experience. Here one must be able to distinguish the experience of an object as being heard, seen, tasted, smelled, or felt. We have a predominant sense through which a parental object becomes knowable and is able to mate with the predominant sense of the other parental object. This results in a link through which the experience of the joined parents in phantasy becomes useable for communication. When this occurs, there is a quality of movement, growth, and experience of emotional interaction. These parental representations are recognizable in the transference as sense representations. This is a form of the sense coding through which the mind locates and retrieves the parents as elements of phantasy.

We have been able to discriminate between identifying the single sense represented in phantasy and to note the unfolding of the phantasy being elaborated. As an example, I will cite sections from an analytic session of a 35-year-old man who demonstrates the phenomenon in question. He states,

> I was annoyed. The people next door were giving a party. The noise came from my bedroom side. I could hear them talking and laughing. I heard actual words. I was falling asleep at eleven o'clock and about twelve there was a huge noise, then they quietened down a bit. It was still noisy and I debated whether I should call on the weekday. I called but it didn't do any good. I took my bedding and put it on the couch in the living room, and then, I became hypersensitive to the noise to see if there was any.

At this point he began rubbing and digging at both eyes very forcefully.

> I had a whole lot of thoughts come as scattered bits of words—I thought they were laughing at keeping me awake. But on simple reflection I knew that was not it. I'm disappointed. I don't feel so good today—I feel so tired but not bad . . . It might have been nice but I wanted to go to sleep. I'm a slow riser, it's sort of a ritual but it's not as much as it used to be. It doesn't seem as if I'm lingering over shaving. This morning I had thoughts of revenge like playing the radio at top volume—I didn't try to control the noise—I turned on the fan—I wasn't considerate of the neighbors—I am already afraid I will be an outcast.

I interpreted to him that, "this was as if a violent war, attack, and desire for revenge was occurring in the room and he was afraid that he would be an outcast here, especially with the separation that occurs over the weekend." [This was a Friday session.] This was his way of talking about parents leaving him out of their life and having a good time while he is put to bed and left out. "You are experiencing the weekend break as if you are being put to bed for the duration of the night in order to allow the adults to have a good time. You resent this and want revenge."

Here, again, he began digging in his eyes and said,

> Yes that is the way I'm feeling . . . Of course there is the actual problem. I'm not really sure what to do about the situation in actuality. It did occur to me to go over there last night but last night I didn't want to get personally involved. My feelings did seem too far out of control to go over and ask them to be quiet. I was just too afraid I'd be laughed at.
>
> ("I think you wanted very much to be up for the action with your parents but felt that if you were to go over there they would certainly feel as if you were a child and they would ridicule and laugh at you—very much in the same way you feel that if you feel personally involved in any way in relation to me then I would reject you as a child and laugh at you.")

He agreed and said,

> I can vaguely remember as a child feeling unhappy when my parents were at a party, wanting to be up for it and also sometimes, if I came into an adult party, everyone would give me a lot of favorable attention and at other times I'd be packed off to bed.

In this example, so far, there is a continual reference to noise, talking, laughing, words, hypersensitivity to sound and retaliation by means of sound—playing the radio at top volume; turning on the fan; making noise—and the resultant fear of punishment or persecution. After the interpretation, the digging response at the eyes involved his taking in information through his ears which led to a visual experience that was indicated by his rubbing in order to avoid the experience of what was seen. He had been able to tell me that at times, when I talked, he noted the presence of visual images and that they were often associated with an experience of itching. If he rubbed his eyes, he felt he could destroy the awareness of the images as they caused pain which he noted to be the result of the experience he had following an interpretation that he felt was accurate. In a way, this could be noted as an attempt to split what is heard from what is seen.

Continuing with the example, the patient states,

> I have this phantasy that everyone around me is suave and sophisticated and there comes to mind a fear of being laughed at. There was a feeling that my parents were deliberately hurting my feelings. The bass came right through the wall. The loud music was so intense I called . . . my girlfriend last night. She had gotten the card and I'd asked her if she wanted to go out. She sounded agreeable and said that she hadn't understood the symbolism but she said she was writing in order to give the relationship more time. We started talking. I felt left out there. On the other hand, when I got back from the hearing, I thought, "If I don't call my girlfriend it'll be questionable." I felt it would be hard to re-establish any relationship, and I thought it would be harder tomorrow when it was the weekend, and I wished someone would do it for me but I knew no one would and I felt somewhat better. It's not realistic to think that my girlfriend is the only woman in the world and maybe I was beginning to do that. I may even meet someone else in the next outing where I met her and I was trying to relate to someone else where our interests don't overlap although I may expect them to be interested almost as a mother which may be unrealistic.

At this point he began digging in his eyes again. I asked him what he was experiencing when he was digging and he said that he had an image but he couldn't remember what it was.

> When I was dating "X" I didn't have a place of my own so I was always at her place.

I mentioned the digging in his eyes and he said, "Yes, it always happens on Friday." I drew attention to the fact that he was feeling as if he could take over the mother and that he had to be very tentative and felt small, obsequious, and fearful of being laughed at. He was talking about the child present in an aspect of his personality at the moment as if over the weekend he was taking revenge and taking over my wife. He then began digging again very intensely over and over and over again, lasting for several minutes. He continued,

> It was going through my head either taking over your wife or yourself or you when I was thinking I wanted mother to be interested in everything I say. It's like the analysis—maybe talking always brings up the feeling of a child talking to a mother. I was pretty apprehensive at the public hearing. I expected angry people to get up and denounce people. Many people were very much in favor of the plan. The administrators of the plan were up at the panel. One lady said it was a bad plan. Someone read a list of all the full-time employees and my name was left off I had asked Miss X and she said I wasn't being dropped. They hired a new person, and I thought they were trying to replace me and leave me out of the organization.

I interpreted that over the weekend he felt that having sex would lead to a new employee, a new baby, and ease him out. Sex was experienced in the form of a public hearing which would result in a new baby who would displace him from the preferred position.

Again, at that point, he had the beginning of a facial tic and digging at his eyes, and he said,

> So that's why I felt so vulnerable, that is why I feel it. I was thinking too something about fear of being thrown out. It was enough like my dream to make me uncomfortable, being left off the list, sitting in an audience, looking up at a stage. The evidence that I'm part of the group is that they have asked me to be there. They didn't ask all the employees, only the ones they thought would make the best showing. The state didn't challenge the employee, they were not in an adversary position.
>
> (I replied that he wasn't certain as to whether I was a friend or an adversary in this particular situation.)

This example shows the definite dissociation between hearing and what is evoked in terms of internal visual phantasy as a result of the interpretation. In this instance a kind of "verbal sex," a primitive sexual representation of contact between two parents, is symbolized in the analytic relationship between analyst and analysand. The connexion between the parents is indicated in terms of a linked pair experienced as leaving him out as the small child. Jealousy is the predominant motive force in the attempt to attack the "parental relationship" substitute. In this example the capacity to link is evident, and the representation of the parental couple is intact. There is considerable evasion of direct contact with the analyst's interventions from within this interaction by a variety of tactics. Delays in responding and seeming agreement with interpretations are noted. The insincerity is noted in terms of not saying what is meant and by rubbing out the visual "free associations" which occurred in response to interpretation.

Avoidance of personal contact is a very common experience in the analytic consulting room. The multitude of contributing factors to the state of lack of contact is far too complex to investigate here. However, the process of conversation, whether analytic or not, is often felt to be a forbidden or pain-inducing phenomenon, especially in the analytic setting. There, the focus of conversation has the direct function of putting the analysand directly in touch with the self and initiates a connexion between split-off aspects of the personality. The establishment of these connections is often fraught with considerable psychic pain initiating powerful resistance (see previous example). The experience of verbal communication relates to primitive infantile dependency situations initially with the mother and subsequently conversation is experienced which cannot be understood by the infant—a reference to being outside of a pair. The infant may experience pain of the absence of need-fulfilling objects' attention, while at the same time recognizing their connectedness through speech.

Primitive jealousy can be the underpinning of the infant's vocalization used as a mode of gaining contact and splitting the focused conversation of the parental pair. Gradually the baby may develop a "controlling" means of capturing attention based on excessive jealousy. Fear, helplessness, and a sense of timeless isolation and pain without boundaries increase the tendency to interrupt external parental contact in order to master painful affect. The voice becomes the means of making connexions as well as breaking them up. To the extent to which infantile primitive experiences have been isolated and split off, the intensity of dependency feelings in direct contact with an object is diminished. The analytic process indeed tends to reapproximate the split which exists not only between mother and father representations, but also between the primary sensory organizational pattern, which is specific in relatedness to each parent.

As if communication then is a variant of an attempt to have a directly linked conversation in such a way as to seem to connect; we believe it is on the way to directness, an attempt at contact. When the parental representations and their primary sensory organizational links are kept split, we have observed a constant conjunction between indirect, as if, distant communication, the lack of dimensionality of experience (analysand), a quality of thinness in the transference, and varying degrees of inability to utilize memory retrieval for information exchanged even within several previous sentences.

The following clinical vignette from a psychoanalytic session with a 27-year-old married woman demonstrates the relationship between memory retrieval and the split between "parental sense representatives."

The patient entered and began to associate about being in a rage at getting a "C" in English. She felt rage at making "stupid" mistakes which she thought centered on being unable to make the distinction between the subject and the object. She continued about the examination and said that she was also in fear about not being able to pass an examination in art history. She was so frustrated because she knew the material very well and recognized the slides used as examples of various paintings. The photographs were being projected on the screen for purposes of written identification but, she said, her verbal thought was interrupted. She could see, but she could not put the words to what she was seeing. She was in a fury. She then remembered a dream. In the dream,

> a *man and a blonde woman were getting ready to have intercourse. She entered* the *room, interrupted and screamed, "you're impotent," and they argued back and forth afterwards. After she left the room, the couple had a violent argument.*

Her association was that she destroyed the relationship between the two of them and certainly destroyed their intercourse. She then remembers her father as not saying much, but being someone she primarily looked at and who had expressive eyes. Her mother was the sort of individual who spoke to her and spent a great deal of time talking to her, though, in fact, did not have a good relationship with the father. She remembers going into the parental bedroom for various sundry excuses but associated that she never heard sounds of intercourse. They were very quiet. She stated: "We were all very quiet." In this instance mother is experienced as the verbal representation and therefore the representation of audition. Her father is the visual. Here is an example of being unable to retrieve memory as a function of not being able to link together the parental representations. Jealousy is clearly seen as the source of difficulty in breaking up the parental representation and breaking up the parental intercourse on a temporary basis.

"To think," the sense link between the parental sensory modalities requires a background of linked parents as a precursor to the phenomenon of thinking. To engage in the thinking process as opposed to having individual thoughts as discrete "sense thoughts" involves a maintenance of the primal scene as represented by a dimensionalization of the parental representations through "common sense." The primal scene is not to be understood as a strictly genital phenomenon, but rather as the primitive experience of the connexion between the parents as experienced by the child through sense representations. This process involves the transformation from oneness (fusion), to twoness, becoming threeness (which has reference to a single object outside of a pair). This is an indication of the capacity to tolerate differences.

In the "inside" state, the markers for this state of mind are extremely subtle, as we have indicated before. The designate "inside" refers to the patient at varying states of psychic fusion (Paul and Carson, 1976; see Chapter 2). We have noted varying stages of psychic fusion to be referenced by specific linguistic forms which relate to varying degrees of completeness of states of psychic fusion. In the more nearly complete state of psychic fusion, *stupid* and *dumb* reference the experience. As separation from the state of psychic fusion begins to develop, the word *weird* appears and upon separation, when the distinction is made between self and object, the word *strange* is often encountered. In the state of mind in which the patient experiences psychic fusion with an object, the general sense of meaning seems to be diminished. When repetitions of the material in the analytic situation occured without the patient seeming to have really grasped or understood and, more importantly, having been able to maintain information in memory is evident and the patient says, "I understand what you say, but I can't remember it at all," one conjecture may be that for a natural retrieval from a memory system there must be associational connections in the matrix between vision and audition so that an expression can be made and one can allow the retrieval of this information just as in music. At least two chords must be stated in order to define a key signature for the ear of the listener. Some process of similar registration—the linkage or convergence of the relatedness of senses—may be necessary in order to allow an impression to be made in an actual memory retrieval system. Two major chords in a particular system will state the actual quality of a particular key in terms of tonality so that the representation of at least two elements fı om a particular family of chords is necessary in order to denote the presence of that particular signature. There may be a similar analogy in the need for representation from at least two senses, i.e. vision and audition; or any other sense such as the close-range senses of touch, taste and smell; or a different kind of experience which will be discussed at a later point.

A 24-year-old male professional student frequently responded affirmatively to analytic interpretations by stating, "Yes, I see what you are saying." At first, one thought nothing of this, but when asked if he was seeing something, he replied that he saw the statement converted directly into printed words that were similar to, but not exactly, that which was stated. He transformed the auditory input to a visual experience that he "saw" outside of himself as if he were viewing a page of typed script. At that point, it became clear that he experienced the analyst's words as if they were entering through his ears and existing through his eyes. This man had a stilted form of speech that seemed baroque. Over years of treatment it had become much more flexible. He was speaking the "written language," which represented a theft of the analyst's words transformed directly into a different sense mode and experienced outside his corporeal self. This fact illuminated the difficulties he had with memory retrieval as well as the ability to work through the material in question since he did not experience the words that he "read" to be contained in his mind. It was as if everything going on in the world had nothing to do with him. He had considerable difficulty with vision in that he had severe strabismus from ages 4 to 7 which was partially connected by surgery involving the extraocular muscles.

The quality of the transference with the patient mentioned above involved the maintenance of an exceedingly abstract use of speech. The abstractions were used concretely, i.e. as a sledgehammer. The subtlety of this particular process depended on the fact that the information transferred in communication was put on an exceedingly high level of abstraction giving the illusion of symbolic communication. The emerging material was not used as symbolic communication, but rather as a means for expelling bits of the personality by means of phantasied ejection or expulsion so that the patient experienced a state of persecutory anxiety denoted by the rapid shift of attention and rapid change to another psychic locale. Attempts at interpretation would always find one off the point in that the patient had already moved very rapidly and subtly to another mental location. One of the hallmarks of this particular transference quality are rapid shifts from place to place and a slipperiness of the interaction in which a patient cannot be "pinned down." Once having called attention to the change in subject, the patient would respond by a shift in time, either to the future or to the past avoiding contact in the present, and might likely distance personal interaction by suddenly interposing another person in phantasy. Very rapid, detailed, active technique is necessary in order to follow patients through the intricacies of their ability to evade direct contact. The patient was capable of changing expelling, or excretory modes from one mental system to another. For example, in the event of his incapacity to utilize his eyes as expelling organs, he shifted to a deep throated cough which was very definitely timed to indicate the near approximation of two sense representations and to prevent the bringing together of the linkages between eye-mother and ear-father, or vice versa. To repeat, subtlety, high levels of abstraction, sleepiness, rapid movements from one locale to another in mental space, the inability to tolerate being confronted, the lack of development of meaning in the therapeutic situation, and the predominance of minute splitting in a sensory mode have been noted in all patients mentioned in this chapter.

With progress in the analytic work and after having achieved the capacity to contain so that there was a relative attenuation of gross projections into resonant objects that stood for aspects of the superego (autocratic, hostile, unforgiving and omnipotent objects), there was a change in the observable patterns of splitting. Rather than a gross attack on the link between patient and analyst, the focus of the split was on the sense links as we have detailed above. Dismantling then occurred when the more gross splitting process had slowed. There was evident a considerable avoidance of any recognition of the distinction between the presence or absence of the analyst as this awareness involving separation might bring on depressive feelings. This particular means of defense is extremely seductive and subtle because there is an impression of the patient's understanding the material. As the patient speaks, one notices his capacity to move and associate with interpretations so that he or she does free associate and the analyst may have the experience of the patient developing a meaningful state of analytic interaction. However, upon closer examination the patient is unable to remember what has been said and, if the patient is perceptive, he will often express the feeling that when directly asked he could not remember from one moment to the next what had actually transpired. Throughout weeks and even years of an analytic process, this incapacity to utilize memory retrieval may be evident. The patient may seem to understand interpretations and even to follow the material at the moment, but no progress is made even though the patient appears to be cooperating in the psychoanalytic process.

This lack of progress in the presence of apparent cooperation may alert us to a possibility that a form of visual expulsion is occurring. One characteristic of some of these patients is their capacity to elaborate dream material in such a way as to evoke an extraordinarily visual and vivid impression in the mind of the analyst. That is, these patients are capable of inducing in one the sense of being able to see the material they elaborate. They speak almost entirely in a visual realm and their capacity to relate is often mediated through the visual channel.

Visual phantasy may be utilized as an isolating mechanism to break off contact and to fix and freeze the material at hand, as in a still photograph, in order to possess it. Because the function of the communication has been to unburden the mind of parts of the personality according to the theory of projective identification, the patient responds to interpretation concretely as if he is being attacked. It is as though the interpretation has been experienced as an action done to the patient rather than having received a symbolic communication. The interpretation of the analyst is experienced concretely, yielding the experience on the part of the patient that something bad has been lodged in him "I can't take it any longer; I have to get out of here." There may follow squirming movements on the couch, a variety of muscular movements, and many rapid complaints one after another. Expulsive movements of all kinds including coughing, sneezing, choking, and feelings of pressure on the bowels as if to defecate have been noted. Thus, the primary mode that has been activated is expulsive, or expelling rather than that of intake. This denotes the inability of the patient to contain the input from the analyst at that point. A reversal of direction of intake to output has occurred. Further, once the sense representatives have been split, either expulsion of the single sense representative, or a shift from one sense to another (such as vision to touch, or hearing to vision) can occur. An example of a patient changing elements of phantasy from an auditory version to a visual version is shown clearly in the next example.

The patient is a 19-year-old male who in this session is describing the manipulations of an amateur radio circuit. He is describing the fact that his radio transmitter has a voice operated relay that activates his antenna to sound and that he has disconnected his antenna from the radio.

> I want to know how much power it's pulling out, and I don't know how much, so if I connect the radio frequency output to a light bulb, I can tell.

> I used a light bulb to develop some kind of impedance matching. I can then tune the transmitter for a dip in plate current and watch for the dip in resonant frequency. That way I am really changing sounds to light. You can take a photo cell and run it through an amplifier and change the voice to light. Then right back to voice. You can make a machine like that for $5.00.
>
> (I interpreted at that point his cheapening the analytic process and shifting his attention away from the vocal interchange that we were having at the moment in attempting to convert it to light.)
>
> He agreed and said, "Yes, too much power burns out the bulb."
>
> (I then interpreted that his attempt to leap from auditory to the visual system was an attempt to avoid a powerful overload.)
>
> That's right. That's right. I can't stand it. This analysis is no good. I can't stand the feelings. I hate it. It'll burn my brain out like I burned out my motorcycle.

(I interpreted that if he attacked on "audio," he felt he was attacked back on "audio.")

He then tried to shift to the visual to avoid contact. I drew his attention to his way of attempting to get a measurement on the outside through a machine, or some sort of electronic device, of how much power, and therefore how much danger there was in a mental burn out. Immediately following, he talked about sexual intercourse being discussed over the citizen band radio which led to a break in the transmission. He experienced conversations about sex as going backwards and forwards at the same time. Here my voice represented the return of the attacked parental split intercourse, or the effect of that in phantasy which the patient is trying to deflect in order to avoid the experience of the intensity of the feelings emerging which are felt as pressure. At the point of interpretation, he developed a headache on the spot so that there is the splitting of visual experience from sound which is meant to clear a channel for use which can bypass the load channel on which the destructive phantasy is occurring. This splitting avoids pain but does not allow thinking. The attempt is, therefore, to try to displace the elements of attack in a particular, singular sense channel and then split it in order to isolate the experience of psychic pain.

A shift in mode from one sense to another may be an indication of the process of making the particular information located in a single sense channel distant from the one in which it has been received. The process of splitting of the parental sense representatives cuts off the awareness of the source of the parental link and also the connection with the analyst who is experienced as the parent in the transference. The patient often feels that even though he has heard the interpretation he has produced it himself.

An example of the subtlety of the visual material put forward in a session may be further elaborated by presenting two dreams of a patient who has been in analysis for four years.

In the first dream of the session, one which was attended with a great deal of anxiety, the patient stated,

> *I was watching a pornographic film. I was watching a man and a woman having intercourse. Then he pulled out, then I'm in, and in the film I grabbed a hold of that man's penis and masturbated it and sucked until he had an orgasm. Then I asked if he would do the same to me; then I woke up.*

The patient associated,

> I had an erection. It just happened. While I repeated the dream it was just like a movie I was telling you about and I could see what you were talking about. In the second dream *I was in a room here and it's dark—like there are no lights on. There is a heavy rain. The rain clouds are outside and I am standing in the middle, and then I have a feeling you are standing right behind me and I turn around. I feel these friendly, warm feelings. The visual image wasn't you. It was maybe you when your hair and beard were darker. You were a lot younger in the dream. I kissed you, and then you said something like, "Lay down on the couch," and we were going to talk. That kiss was saying goodbye to Judy. I felt this abandoned, hurt feeling that there was no good. I was asking you, "Where do I find purpose and meaning?" You said, "Go to church." I was scared and I woke up in the old way.*

He associated,

> What left me in the other world was I wasn't sure it happened or whether I had taken it from the dream, or whether the dream was here, but as I was talking I saw it, and I understand now why I had so much trouble remem-

> bering. I think my memory is vision, or vision is my memory. Or, why it was so difficult for me to repeat back what someone has said or hold it in long enough to keep it, say in a set of class notes. It's too damn dangerous. I think for me sound is sexual, and it feels painful. I can't stand it. The feeling of not being able to hold in sound without anxiety makes me so upset that I can't tolerate it.

The theory of attacks on linking as a means of preventing the experience of jealousy and/or envy has been discussed by Bion (1967). In this example, we have a clear representation in a dream in which there is interruption of the intercourse between the parents, a situation in which there is an analogy between the psychoanalytic situation and a sexual situation. The patient feels that he is taking in something from the psychoanalytic penis which is inseminating him and is experienced as occurring in relation to sound (speech). The inseminating experience seems to be occurring through the ears or the auditory senses and is also felt to be so dangerous that it must be evacuated out through the eyes in phantasy in the form of a dream which is seen as it is told. This is a way of breaking the intercourse between the seminal homosexual relationship between the father and the child—brought about from a phantasy utilizing auditory means—and enables the child, the patient in this regard, to "get in" to the dream itself. The patient puts forward the dream which is seen outside of him as a hallucinatory experience and feels himself to be entering the dream as mother's representative. (In this patient, mother was experienced as predominantly visual.)

As a further example of the use of dissociating one sense from another, we will consider a typical experience of an analysand who masks feelings with his voice. He puts forward a well-tempered, modulated, gentle quality which has the feel of smoothness without any obvious hard-edged quality that one would ordinarily associate with social insincerity. Statements such as, "I'm having the thought, 'I hate you'" or, "I'd like to hit you" are reported as if the word presentation of the thoughts was emerging without any affective intensity. There is further distancing from direct communication by the attitude of the patient's representing "his state of mind" for the purpose of "helping the analysis." His anxiety often begins to betray itself by his acknowledgement of "a feeling of anxiety," his nose will seem to "stuff" within seconds, and there will be a quick removal of his glasses attended by a vigorous knuckle-digging motion of hand in orbit (eye socket) with a powerful intensity and vigorousness.

When this sequence is brought to his attention, he responds by acknowledging a powerful itching sensation which required the knuckle-digging "scratching." This sequence is stereotyped and puts a stop to further associations in the domain of the subject under consideration. An abrupt switch of direction, time, and subject ensues at great speed. This is attended by a hardness and clipped, bitten-off quality in the voice which has the effect of a "cutting" feeling.

Each element within this episode may be noted to have coded meaning. Elements associated with vision are the removal of glasses, digging, and the sensation of itching. As these symptoms become apparent, the presence of these elements in various forms are noted in other patients and in everyday life. Movements include intense pressure on the "globes," stated change in the retinal pattern produced by the digging, and in a series of light flashes as if on an internal screen. Often there will be described dimly colored patterns or dots which change with the knuckle-digging motions. Characteristically, this eye scratching may be bilateral and often may require long periods of rubbing from seconds to minutes in severe episodes. The person will usually "rub his eyes" until they are quite inflamed. We are postulating this experience of ablation of phantasy attached to the visual sense to be a form of mental attack on the links between senses, one of which is visual. Meltzer (1975) has referred to this process in his study on autism as "dismantling." We are postulating this mental attack on linkage to represent not only a dedimensionalizing experience, but also to represent an insidious form of stopping the development of the analytic evolving experience.

There is a very strong association of this pattern to the subject of oedipal murder in phantasy. Gross attacking hostility in conscious form may be noted although more frequently subtle, insidious attacks which reduce to murder are evident. Generally the attacks are "silent" in that they give the quality of being so disguised that they effectively obscure any violence. The transference quality has the feeling of a *fait accompli* where it is as if there was no possibility of any interchange which could have even vague meaning. This may lead to feelings in the analyst of an experience of uselessness and increasing anxiety. There is an evolution of a catastrophic situation which leads to a fragmentation of thinking and scattering with ensuing suspiciousness and distancing on the part of the patient. At first this may appear to be a sudden silence, a slight confusional state which will be passed off. Further investigation may yield the following sequence:

1. There are clear elements of the oedipal myth scattered in the preceding material, such as references to blindness, exile, and murder itself. Both parricide and infanticide show up at times, with different

outcomes.

2. There is a quality of nonverbalized action present in the session.
3. The process becomes more concrete as it proceeds. Phantasied infanticide leads to a terror of anything which forms anew, no matter on what level of abstraction.

Parricide allows for greater flexibility and excursion of phantasy. Anxiety and depression usually accompany parricide. The future is represented, but is feared. The unknown is treated as if it were known to be frightening. Psychic movement has a backward quality. The direction towards desired objects of need are rapidly reversed.

There are clear rhythm patterns of the evolution of phantasy within a period after one of the forms of oedipal mental murder. A turbulence follows parricide with increasing velocity of speech, intensity of effect, and there is development of consciously felt anxiety. High speed thinking, with increasing breaks in rhythm and rapid stops, characterize the feel.

One might consider the splitting of parental sense representatives as a means to maintain the state of psychic fusion by avoiding the correlation of information from incoming sense data which would allow for the perception and separation from an object, this allowing it independence. By contrast, the question arises, "How does a child make the distinction between self and not self?" The senses are utilized to discover this distinction. We speculate that when the senses are used to attack the links between parents fusion is maintained. But, as the attacks are diminished, further opportunity exists to make the distinction between self and not self.

The sense representatives which are dismantled in order to break a linkage between mother and father representations appear no longer able at that moment to serve as a tool for making the distinction between self and not self, as further resolution of fusion becomes hampered. Specific senses are identified as referencing to the experience of distance from the primary object, such as vision and hearing (long range) as opposed to touch, taste (short range) and smell (mid range), and come to lead to distinctions between self and not self by means of reversing the direction of the key sense experiences which define the distinction, the process of psychological differentiation can be reversed in phantasy. In doing so, the sense experience which would have been used to define a distinction is no longer available for recombination within the boundaries through which effective linking must occur in order to generate an evolving thinking process. Hence, the representative senses involved are "jammed" and the information which would have been used for linking is no longer available for use in forming the basis for an evolving thought process. The existence of this jamming indicates a point of distinction between the state of psychic fusion and the emergence of the earliest oedipal situation as mediated by sensory integrative experience.

The sense modality used to locate the parent in the state of distinction may not necessarily be the same modality used to communicate with the parent or the therapist in the transference.

We have attempted to show how the senses can be represented in phantasy and how specific predominant senses can represent the parents. At the earliest level of mind, referenced to "outside," the object forms via an amalgamation of sensory experience. The convergence of relatedness between sense representatives leads to the experience of dimensionality. We are postulating that the object representation is a secondary derivative of the senses. The experience of dimension varies as a function of range. That is, if close range senses are utilized at long range experience and phantasy, the patient's experiences of distance and perception of dimension are altered from clarity to "mental myopia." The converse is also noted when long range senses are utilized at short range. The interplay of sensory representations in phantasy shift mental boundaries and thereby alter psychological meaning not only by changing the dimensions of internal space, but by altering the experience of dimension of the mental objects in relation to boundaries. Further, we have confirmed Meltzer's description of dismantling and extended the concept to reference to the phenomenon of mental murder and memory retrieval.

Summary

In this chapter, we explore the means by which the senses are represented in phantasy and how specific senses may represent the parents. The theory that the parental intercourse is a model for instigation of the thinking process by linking each parent to a separate sense modality is developed. The linkage of primitive sense data in organized coded form leads to the experience of dimension. The organization of sense representatives in phantasy shift mental boundaries and thereby alter psychological meaning not only by changing the dimension of internal space, but by altering the experience of dimension of the mental objects in relation to boundaries.

Nonverbal aspects of the parricidal and infanticidal transference are explored as a function of the oedipal myth. Splitting of the sense representatives as a variant of attacks on linking are directly related to difficulties in memory retrieval.

Chapter 4

A Mental Atlas of the Process of Psychological Birth

In his *Inhibitions, Symptoms and Anxiety* (1926), Freud was concerned not only with the relations between anxiety and symptom formation, but with certain aspects of the process of birth which had been primarily introduced by Otto Rank's consideration of the birth trauma. Rank (1929) was concerned, as was Freud, not with the elements of a birth process as revealed by the analysis of unconscious phantasy, but rather with the "traumatic" aspects of birth in relation to the development of a theory of anxiety. It is clear, however, that Freud was aware of exceedingly primitive mnemic residues which could be ascribed to birth traumata, but was critical of Rank's attempt to simplify the theory of anxiety to a singular aetiology in the birth trauma.

> Anxiety is not newly created in regression, it is reproduced as an affective state in accordance with an already existing mnemic image. If we go further and enquire into the origin of that anxiety—and of affects in general—we shall be leaving the realm of pure psychology and entering the borderland of physiology. Affective states have become incorporated in the mind as precipitates of primeval traumatic experiences and when a similar situation occurs they are revived like mnemic symbols (p. 93).

He continues,

> We cannot possibly suppose that the fetus has any sort of knowledge that there is a possibility of its life being destroyed. It can only be aware of some vast disturbance in the economy of its narcissistic libido. Large sums of excitation crowd in on it giving rise to new feelings of un-pleasure and some organs acquire an increased cathexis, thus foreshadowing the object's cathexis that will soon set in. What elements in all this will be made use of

> as the sign of a danger situation? It is easy to say that the baby will repeat its affect of anxiety in every situation that recalls the event of birth. The important thing to know *is "what recalls the event and what is it that is recalled"* (p. 135).

It is in reference to this last point that I wish to begin the consideration of how we can recognize elements of these "primeval" mnemic residues which are preverbal and contained in sense channels which are unrecognizable to ordinary communication. I wish to elaborate certain connections between a life which I believe is a representation of a prenatal experience and the postnatal world taking as a point of inspiration Freud's (1926) statement, "There is much more continuity between intrauterine life and earliest infancy than the impressive caesura of the act of birth allows us to believe" (p. 138).

We are familiar with the experience of being exposed to certain aspects of obsessional "thinking" which has a cyclic quality. There is no forward motion of a train of thought developed on a "track."

The individual feels subjected to "painful thoughts" or rather thoughts which cannot be thought through and are associated with severe mental pain more or less depending upon the content. Patients will refer to "dwelling" on their thoughts, "ruminating," "worrying," and mean a repetitive circularity which continues and is associated with increasing emotional pain. This "pain" is so important that one realizes that a good deal of modern drug habituation to tranquilizers, sleeping medications and alcohol addiction results from attempts to reduce or abate the pain. The thought cycle may take a variety of forms but several definable features can be noted: repetitive quality, lack of progression to a higher level of abstraction, lack of linking capacity, concreteness, peremptory quality, a tendency to impel to action, and profound intrusiveness. This last point is of extreme importance as patients often begin to anticipate with dread the sudden intrusion of the painful pattern of thoughts which then "think" them or rather control their minds such that little else is felt to occur. When patients experience these "thoughts," they complain often of insomnia and complain that they cannot stop the process. An action is necessary in order to put a stop to this state of mind which may be any of a variety from self-induced narcosis to physical violence. One often hears the expression, "I can't get these thoughts off my mind," "they won't leave me alone," etc. The "thoughts" are felt to possess the thinker and often are felt to be experienced as holding or grasping tenaciously. This process is accompanied frequently by anxiety and agitation.

Attempts are made at this time to disburden the mind of these unpleasant experiences which frequently results in massive projective identification (Klein, 1957; Bion, 1962).

I have noted in several patients powerful attempts to put a stop to my communications at certain key points in a session as they are felt in advance to be quite dangerous and are defended against with great force. These patients behave as though any further communication would certainly lead to a catastrophe and instigate something which would seem to be irrevocable.

Mrs. X, a 47-year-old mother of two, suffers an incapacity to work, extreme anxiety, marked agitation, alcoholism and extreme obesity. She has marked insomnia and experiences her "thoughts" as visual images of varied content but "knows" that there are certain forms of these thoughts which are far too dangerous to verbalize. Sometimes she feels that if she were to "say what she sees," whatever it is would "happen" and resolutely refuses at that point to continue. She is aware of categories of thought which she divides into categories such as "I'm too tired to talk about them," "I can only talk about them sometimes," and "These can *never* be verbalized." When these "thoughts" emerge into her conscious mind, she can be seen to shudder and often begins to weep uncontrollably. She squirms on the couch and has intense pain. No attempt at interpretation has been successful in leading to any further flow of material at these times. Often she is mute and if an interpretation is "close to the mark," she will become enraged and has an attitude that states that I don't realize what I could do to her if in fact I were to continue. At that time I am felt to be stupid or utterly cruel. "How could you?" is her response, which may remain weeks to months in her mind. She is virtually unable to let go of the phantasy that I may have induced this response.

This woman, highly articulate, well-educated, and a skilled writer, realizes that these episodes involve intense superstition, understands the massive degree of irrationality she experiences and is utterly ashamed of her inability to dare to cooperate under these circumstances. At these times she is in profound despair, utterly hopeless and convinced that nothing she nor I can do will produce a change. She frequently calls herself stupid and dumb with intense force, and describes herself as a perpetual "fool." She utilizes these epithets as a means of producing psychic closure and the flow of material stops abruptly. She is then "caught between," as it were, her realization that her despair stems from her failure and inability to cooperate, and her intense fear that cooperation will lead to catastrophe. She is functionally unable to make distinctions in time. The past, present, and future are confused, and she predicts the future entirely based on her past despair, which compounds the hopelessness.

This is quite similar to the "no exit" situation which Sartre depicts in his play. She is "stuck" as she describes and portrays very well the concept of therapeutic impasse.

At this mental location she typically states, "There is no point to this; I can't see the point in continuing, but I'm too terrified not to come to analysis." One might ask: Why is she "stuck"? Where is she "stuck"? or What is the point she is seeking?

An important analytic "fact" is evidenced in that these attempts at closure are most obvious at the end of the session, the end of the week, and holidays. When this patient gets up, she complains of a feeling of dizziness and profound disorientation and often remains in the exit portion of the office for several minutes after leaving the consulting room. The patient demonstrates an obstruction in her thinking process in that she cannot come to the "point" she is attempting to reach as a result of what she feels is a "blanking" of her mind. Often she feels there is no point either in what I say or what she thinks. She is never sure whether she "really" thinks what she says, and makes reference to the possibility that even though she might not mean it to be, she could be fabricating parts of the material. She does not lie as far as she can tell, but neither is she certain that what she says is the truth.

I have noted this "doubt" of the truth of her narrative to occur subsequent to her having stopped the flow of her speech. After this "stop," there is often a change of vocal tone which I can notice, followed by her "doubt" of the truth of what she says. This patient states and has demonstrated that this process is very different from purposive lying, as she would simply refuse to talk consciously which has been amply demonstrated throughout the analysis.

Bion (1970) distinguishes between true thoughts and lies, in that "a thinker is logically necessary for the lie but not for the true thought" (p. 102). He continues, "The lie and the true thought are inseparable. The thinker is of no consequence to the truth, but the truth is logically necessary to the thinker" (p. 103). Further,

> The lie gains existence by virtue of the epistemologically prior existence of the liar . . . Whether the thoughts are entertained or not is of significance to the thinker but not to the truth. If entertained, they are conducive to

mental health; if not, they initiate disturbance (p. 103).

The process of emergence of thoughts inseparable from the thinker as a function of the lie then must be considered in the clinical description given above. Are the thoughts we are referring to emerging "true" thoughts which seem to erupt spontaneously from the infinite Galactic void of mental space which create a disturbance associated with their arrival? Psychoanalytic evidence suggests that the means by which these "thoughts" are processed are inadequate to transform them to thinking the thought through. These thoughts are then subject to ejection in phantasy since the "mind" of the patient in question has not the equipment for effective transformation of thought. One distinction between the lie and true thought in Bion's terms may relate to the difference between "conjury or invention" versus spontaneous emergence without effort. In the analytic session, there is a difference between the "thought" emerging through directly, and the divergent pathway of the thought going around an obstruction. The former affords penetration to awareness, while the divergent route is essentially an evasion. One version of the "lie" then in this context may refer to this divergent pathway as an evasion.

To return to the case being considered . . . in her fourth year of treatment she dreamed that she was in an autopsy room watching the end of a postmortem which then transformed into an embalming scene. She saw the circulatory hookup and as the process was begun, she awakened screaming from her dream but could not shake off the hideous sensation of being flooded and engorged with fluid as the embalming began. She stated she could feel the fluid flooding every element of her being and at that time had a resurgence of a previous active symptom, a choking phobia which had been intensely limiting of her activities.

Phantasizing being inside mother immediately preceded this dramatic example taking the form of her replicating in the transference relationship between herself and myself the phantasy of the ability to know everything I was thinking, what I would interpret next, and so forth. She has been dominated by these forms of omniscience especially developed in her relation to her mother as a model. Mother was described as intensely critical with an unerring eye for the perception of the bad. The patient's history suggests a mother who was unable to contain her child's infantile anxieties and responded by abrupt separation. My patient learned to "track" and telemeter mother's mental meanderings in order to ward off the abrupt experience of pain upon intense, scathing criticism.

The themes of crisis, criticism, and hypocrisy were evident not only in this patient's analysis but in the analyses of each of the eight patients of this type with whom I have had experience.

Crisis in Greek means to separate, whereas *criticism* has as a main definition the process of distinction which also is associated with separation. *Hypocrisy*, I reasoned, means, literally, below criticism or beneath the divide and refers to not making a distinction with a pejorative connotation. These themes revolve around phantasies associated with the prenatal state-hypocrisy with cowardly nondistinction and crisis especially with the experience of impending psychological birth. Criticism employed in a destructive hostile manner can be seen by the moral approach to make the boundary between the inside and outside.

The patient has been a chronic alcoholic who is "soused," in her own terms, and thus far has been unable to stop. She drinks to stop separation anxiety and shows what could be interpreted as excessive greed noted by her extraordinary anxiety. In the dream mentioned above, she associated to drinking and being "pickled," but there were clear references to prenatal experience. Greed seems to me to be a moral term and, although descriptive, has a profoundly negative connotation. Is the extreme sensitivity of a quasifetal-infantile state of mind still operating on the model, or a placental feed a mental state which can brook no separation from a continuously feeding object another way of describing greed? Are we witnessing the phenotype of a primitive, perhaps fetal, mental state in the adult world? In this way, the presence of the moral approach denoted by the transition in linguistic usage from descriptive-phenomenological to moralistic quality of language is a marker for the appearance of the gap between pre- and post-natal experience. This concept bears close relation to addictive states, as well as the general conception of narcissism which will be explored in other works (Paul, 1989, 1997; see Chapters 8, 9).

To return to Mrs. X's dream, it is possible to consider it as a representation of a prenatal experience having achieved representation associated with a severely dysphoric state. Upon interpretation of this dream, the patient questioned her mother and discovered that she indeed had a toxemia of pregnancy which was exacerbated just prior to birth.

Another patient likened his relationship to the analyst to an experience with a renal dialysis machine without which he could not live.

A series of phenomena, both nonverbal and verbal, have become significant across a group of at least eight patients who have severe narcissistic disorders.

1. The consulting room is felt to be markedly different from the external world. Disorientation and/or severe dizziness often accompany entering and/or leaving. Upon entering, often the patient avoids contact with me directly and often finds great difficulty leaving. In phantasy, the consulting room is experienced as "inside the mother's body." Often I am incidental or mostly felt not to be present.

2. These patients show evidence of long-standing, rather complete projective identification and show extreme sensitivities to the perception of heat and cold as a constant. By projective identification, I mean to convey a quality of deep psychic fusion with an internal phantasy of being-in-the-mother's body. This state of mind is predominant and rather fixed, any deviation from which is immediately attended by a sense of impending catastrophe. This is to be distinguished from an oscillating quality in which other patients move in and out of a state of being "inside." The patients experiencing projective identification behave as though they were hermetically sealed in a world never to be exposed to the air. One such patient in previous analysis for twenty years wore long winter underwear at all times to protect himself from the "cold" which he "might" experience. Upon successful interpretation of a state of psychic fusion with "mother's" body, the patient will suddenly note the presence of sudden "cold." A rapid change in temperature within a split second of the interpretation is experienced, and piloerection is grossly observable as an accompanying phenomenon. Two of these patients have given histories of a special supersensitivity to cold, in that they state that they can distinguish between one degree Fahrenheit up or down and talk about temperature very frequently as a general analytic theme.

In both patients who are specifically sensitive to cold, neither has had any demonstrable physiologic reason and both have had repeated, thorough endocrinologic studies. In addition, both are subject to frequent "colds" and the "flu," which makes them extremely wary of draughts, night air, etc.

3. Interpretation of the stages of projective states leads very rapidly to changes in the perception of sound, temperature, visual acuity, visual clarity, and will produce disorientation and dizziness, often with severe transitory vertigo as the boundary between inside and outside is crossed in phantasy. Sudden changes in perception then signal the

shift from inside to outside, and vice versa. Warmth, stuffiness, and an uncomfortably enclosed sensation are well-known markers for the "inside" experience. The dizziness and disorientation distinguish a level of primitiveness which links to the representation in phantasy of the birth process. In my experience, the shift in perception of temperature and the sudden onset of dizziness are the most reliable indicators of a change in state of mind which related directly to the experience of birth.

4. Sudden onset of headache, often frontal and rhythmically pounding, is an associated phenomenon noted in the context of this change in state of mind from inside to outside. Pain of a band-like pressure quality across the forehead and usually bilaterally symmetrical is a common finding. If the pressure is not felt intrinsically, often the patient will press hands quite forcibly against the forehead and the top of the head associated with phantasies of moving back from outside to inside. The pounding headache does not have a vascular periodicity and is not regular or in synchrony with the heartbeat, but occurs as an indefinite, unpleasant sensation occurring "within the head" at a frequency of several times a minute. The force of speech in rhythmical patterns with a periodic repetitiveness may be noted clearly to precede the actual physical sensation even though the pounding speech pattern may exist without the physical quality and vice versa.

5. A sensation of "pressure" usually felt about the head is frequently associated with a stoppage of the "sinuses" and has been noted in several patients as "waves" over the body passing from the head to the feet in rhythmic force. Often this pressure sensation and upper respiratory partial obstruction is associated with the patient putting at least a temporary end to communication and is noted to be a form of grammatical "period." This is a transitional phase from inside to outside and is often accompanied by terror-panic. I have noted that at this point there is associated a profound splitting of sense modalities, for example hearing from vision which seems to uncouple the transitional process of movement in psychic space (Paul and Carson, 1980; see Chapter 3).

The respiratory phenomena include in some patients a sudden gasping for air or in smokers the holding of smoke inside their lungs to the point of pain. Upon questioning, the internal "outlining" of the respiratory passages so that the internal aspects of the lungs could be felt was the salient feature in several patients, not the feeling of air hunger. Breathing is often "held" fixed for long pauses during which all activity stops and the consulting room atmosphere "feels" dead. Profound tightening of the throat musculature and intense fear of choking may ensue in selected cases.

6. In a single case of this type I noted the presence of oedema which had been diagnosed as idiopathic associated with phantasies of fusion with the mother's body, which specifically and progressively remitted upon interpretation of these phantasies. This analysand has been addicted to a powerful diuretic for a number of years which she took for "depression."

I shall present an additional case example to demonstrate a series of phenomena which are important for the development of understanding of the preverbal phenomena linked to elements of the postulated pre-birth and birth experience.

As the patient enters, she hunches and averts her eyes so as to avoid any emotional connection between us. She moves to the couch and sits on the edge and settles for a moment as if in deep reflection. Silently she swivels toward me with her body maintaining a downcast eyes-half-shut-mien. Suddenly her head snaps to a position on direct confrontation to mine and glares. This movement is stereotyped and evokes a quality of tension which is so powerful that she quickly averts her eyes and communication is at a halt. It is as if the scene has been set for expectation of an emotional explosion which has been the usual sequel for the past two years. A gradually increasing crescendo of complaining begins in a demanding, whining voice which has a piercing resonance. The rhythm picks up speed as does the intensity although the volume remains approximately the same. Attempts at interpretation even after ten minutes or longer of steady repetition are ignored, cut off, and attempts are made to stop the analyst's speech. Any attempt to persevere meets with an increase of voice force and intensity meant to keep the analyst's position fixed to silence. The grating quality picks up again with increasing repetitiveness and intensity which fills the consulting room with a tension that is palpable both in patient and analyst. I am aware of an increasing sense of intense pain which evokes in me an experience of emotionally wanting to shut down, or yields a powerful quality of annoyance and isolation, and suddenly I become aware of hatred which threatens to lead to action. I have noticed a desire to strike out, to shout her down, to get rid of her in any way possible. Introspection upon this phenomenon reveals the pattern of vocal qualities mentioned above, brought forward in a rhythmical, repetitive, increasing crescendo grating which evokes intense feelings in the analyst.

The content of the material continually has to do with expectations of disaster, and how nothing can help her. She feels trapped, encocooned, irrevocably damaged; time has passed her by; the future will bring only disaster and terror. She wonders what will she do, and feels she must do something, as I or no one else can help her return from having reached the point of violence she intuits. Then as if she were at the end of a cadenza, she returns to the beginning again, "D.C. al Fine," with increasing percussiveness, so that the verbal material is more felt than heard, and the piercing resonance mentioned above increases. This I have named "repetition percussion," as it heralds the experience which, if continued, leads to blinding dizziness, loss of orientation in space, terror, and such intense blaming hatred that she avows that mere contact with me has produced the experience which is so frightening she cannot continue it and yet cannot stop until either she has reached a limit at which point the dysphoric state will be interrupted by a violent mental event signaled by the sudden presence of dizziness.

In the second year a specific timing of these rhythmic patterns began to emerge. When she would be expecting her menses, which were highly irregular and usually delayed often by two to three weeks, she would experience increasing irritability, intense frustration about minor issues and would begin the haranguing diatribe mentioned above, leave the session in utter frustration, usually weaving and staggering out the door after having almost lurched into me, which was always out of her way to do. She would say, "I don't know where I am," appear to be drugged, linger at the exit, and finally leave in disgust after having attempted to instill me with a sense of my utter cruelty. The dizziness was so severe, there was question as to her ability to walk. She would apologize about "what I am doing to you," but persist with repeated phone calls two to three times an evening during the week before a period. She had dreams of herself as a shrimp exposed to the world without a shell and in utter danger. During this period she had on her own recognizance a complete medico-endocrinologic study including a neurological workup, which was negative. She was terrified that she was hemorrhaging to death although she had awareness that her menstrual flow was within her usual limits. Similar events such as these gave rise to her breaks from treatment with two other analysts, both of whom had treated her five years each.

Associated with these intense "attacks" she would "look for a fight" with fellow employees, negate anyone who attempted to approach her, and demonstrated especial hatred for her mother, whom she could not forgive for giving birth to her. She had lost many jobs because of this behavior and stated that both her previous analysts terminated treatment with her because of it. It was only a matter of time before I would do the same because she felt that she was at an "impasse" which would not "give." Either she would die, end up in an institution, or I would be severely damaged, according to her.

It became increasingly evident that there was a sharp contrast between her feeling in the room the "instant" she entered compared with her experience outside. She felt she could be relatively calm, but take one look at me and be struck with hatred, confusion, and gradual numbness. I interpreted to her that her menstrual periods were experienced as if she were giving birth to a damaged baby which had been pounding against the uterine wall again and again attempting to emerge, but at an impasse. Her repeated rhythmical attempts to break out were repetitious of her experience at birth which led to her mother's exhaustion and the patient's increasing sense of "terror." These interpretations over a period of several months appeared to "take" and the violence diminished although aspects of the above experience were repeated with every period. She discovered upon questioning her mother that such an event as reconstructed analytically actually did occur with her mother developing a secondary uterine inertia which resulted in caesarian section. Thus the pounding rhythm, the bloody phantasies of damaged children, parts of the body scattered over the streets, phantasies of violent accidents transforming to the shrimp dreams, and sudden confusion and disorientation corresponded to the particular discrete events associated with parturition.

The transition from a watery environment to a gaseous medium has been studied in great detail by embryologists. Anatomical and physiologic adaptations to the sudden shift from water to air involve massive changes in circulatory dynamics as the umbilical cord is clamped with the well-known closure of the shunt through the foramen ovale and the subsequent sudden initiation of flow through the respiratory circuit which had been dormant. As the amniotic membranes rupture the pressure of the amniotic fluid which had suspended the fetus in flotation suddenly decreases, although while in utero the fetus must be subject to an experience of increased pressure relatively evenly distributed over its body through direct contact. Although we do not know directly, the fetus may experience sensations received from the mother's body either by direct approximation (i.e., uterine contractions) or through her circulatory system via the placenta. It is entirely likely that affective states such as anxiety which are mediated by humoral agents (i.e., epinephrine) reach the fetus as a passive recipient. Recent studies with premature infants have suggested that the fetus perceives sound in-utero coming from borborygmi and from the maternal circulatory system. Sound travels four times faster in water than in air and would depend for its reception upon the fetus being able to transduce the "pressure waves" of sound in a fluid medium to a form of auditory trace.

Bion (1975) has reminded us that if one closes one's eyes, pressure on the globes will result in seeing lights. This can be confirmed by the reader.

Thus it is likely that some form of input from outside the fetus' anatomy comes in and is received through a form of vision and hearing, but mediated through a pressure modality. This feature of sensory input via a pressure system may be an important reference for the "dating" of the experience of pressure when it becomes an important analytic theme.

With the birth process in physical form, the blood flow is cut off from the mother and the fetus must undergo a rapid shift from a gill-like form of respiration to the use of the lungs. The external fluid pressure on the skin is suddenly reduced and the organs of sensation from the skin to olfaction, vision, and hearing must undergo a fundamental change in the threshold of stimulation. The fetus as it is born is suddenly subjected to intensities of sound, light, temperature, and touch, which is entirely different from its intrauterine experience.

Even though the reader is familiar with the elements of the birth process, consideration of each of the issues mentioned above shows that nothing less than a major stage in evolution which required millennia in the history of phylogeny occurs regularly with every human birth in a matter of seconds.

I have noted a number of unchanging phrases in current linguistic usage that refer to the phases of the transitional process from inside the mother in phantasy to birth (Paul and Carson, 1976; see Chapter 2).

The experience of psychic movement toward psychological birth is attended by what seems to be severe mental pain. Terror and severe intense anxiety are frequently described. "I can't make ends meet," "I'm under extreme pressure," "I'm up against the wall," "I've gotten in over my head," are frequent references to the instigation of the shift to the outside. In the intermediate process, one frequently hears, "I'm out on a limb,"

"I've over-extended myself." References to the outside state include vertigo, "I'm out in the cold," etc. The experience of separation from an object which is used as though it were expected to be placental is extremely traumatic. The term placental-object describes the nature of the form of psychic attachment to the analyst and delineates the expectations which are placed upon him by the patient. Bion (1967) has described psychotic transference as "thin and tenacious." These patients show a similar tenacity and adhesiveness. The patients conform in description to the grown-up version of the children described by Meltzer *et al.* (1975) in their *Explorations in Autism.* The patient feels he cannot afford to allow the analyst time separately simply because he will die if separated. He feels "cut off," "ripped off," as in umbilical cord and placenta and cannot tolerate independent existence without the presence of a nourishing object.

These patients treat the analyst as if he were present only in a very undifferentiated form. They experience the analysis as a place to be, but do not have a conception of taking something in. A profound hatred is evidenced for anything which reminds them of the feeding situation. Two of these patients gave histories of failure to thrive in infancy and one had severe celiac disease associated with chronic diarrhea from earliest infancy through the age of one-and-one-half years. Severe colic was evidenced in three others, lasting a full year with marked inability to sleep, and they gave histories of pronounced screaming throughout the night which could only be soothed by the presence of a parent rocking them through the night. They evidence a wish to be held about which they are very guarded and interpret the analyst's intervention as an attempt to force feed them which they ward off as if a catastrophe would occur if they were to listen or try to understand. If the patients do listen, they experience "pressure," feel "pressured," and there is a sudden ushering in of a delinking process so that the analyst's constructions are rendered meaningless. This "pressure" has similarity to the patients' experience when mentally located in utero just prior to birth in phantasy. It is almost as if any intake would destroy their delusion of being in a state of uterine sanctuary.

We do not have the methodology to specifically demonstrate the exact developmental links of intrauterine life in symbolic form through the development of infancy and childhood which would satisfy the scrutiny of strict scientific validation. How does the fetus and even the infant "remember" the events described above? The fetus and infant would have to be capable of registering the experience in memory and then retrieve it in a symbolic form enough to even verbalize the phantasies as have been described. The development of symbolic communicative skill does not develop at least until 12-18 months (Mahler, 1968), which then leaves us with a mystery. It is convenient, as many including myself have done, to deny prematurely the validity of such formulations. If, however, when the child gains communicative skills, the verbal forms which are linked to invariant deep structural patterns (Chomsky, 1957, 1968) are capable of containing the code locked in the soma, the succeeding development of complexity of language better enables the person to transcribe and translate a primitive language which requires the symbol for further transformation. The development of language would then bridge the gap between a primitive somatic experiential language and what we understand as symbolic phantasy. That verbal forms can be utilized for transcribing primitive body language after birth has already been amply demonstrated by Melanie Klein (1961) and extended by Hanna Segal (1956) in her description of the development of the symbolic equation. I mean to extend these important discoveries to include an even more primitive state in order to postulate the existence of a form of experience in utero which is registered by the fetus and which is capable of translation at a later time into a symbolic form.

Further, Mrs. Klein (1970) describes "phantasied onslaughts on the mother following two main kinds: one is the predominantly oral impulse to suck dry, bite up, scoop out and rob the mother's body of its good contents. The other line of attack derives from the anal and urethral impulses and implies expelling dangerous substances (excrements) out of the self and into the mother." She continues, "These excrements and bad parts of the self are meant not only to injure, but also to control and to take possession of the object" (p. 300). In her pioneering description of projective and introjective mechanisms, she defined the earliest object relations after birth and made mention briefly of the sources of primary anxiety as being related to the trauma of birth (Klein, M., 1952). In the above description, it appears to me that the attempts to forcefully gain nutrients and locate waste in the maternal object not only relate to oral and anal aggressive phantasies, but also relate to the attempt to maintain a functioning placenta as a primary expectation which has never been worked through. In the intrauterine state, there is no oral feeding or anal excretion as all of these functions are perfectly handled by the placenta as intermediary between the mother and fetus. Might this not relate to the frequent expectations of perfection rigidly maintained in schizoid patients? Birth is then literally a rip-off (as defined in current parlance) which is experienced as a violent robbery, battery, and attempted murder on the part of the mother and vice versa.

A frequent finding in these patients has been a form of drug addiction or habituation from alcohol through hallucinogens. The drug is phantasied to put them in touch with the experience of being inside a mother by means of taking a psychoactive agent which can be "felt" to act within them. A striking finding has been the lack of specificity of the drug used for the most part as long as the experience of the "feel" of the drug acting inside them is evident (Paul, 1997; see Chapter 10). Regardless of major pharmacologic differences in the drugs utilized, several patients described no ability to discriminate between these drugs even those thought to be widely different in activity on a spectrum between alcohol, barbiturates, and tranquilizers on the one hand and stimulants on the other. The experience they seek in common is the "rush" from the perception of the feel of the drugs beginning to take effect and the dose is self-adjusted until this experience is reached. The experience of diminution of anxiety or the ablation of the "birth" symptoms of pressure, etc., is not the main target, but rather the maintenance of a feeling of something active inside them which they can control. Even if on a very potent drug, such as Ritalin or amphetamine in relative naive users, the effect on the mental process is denied unless they can continue to feel the "rush" and then continue to increase the dose until "psychological tolerance" is reached.

Often several patients have been in various states of obvious narcosis, but have denied perceiving any such state of mind unless the drug's activity is felt as the driving force of the "rush." Within the drug culture, a very clear discrimination is made between those habitués who use drugs orally versus those who "mainline" or inject by vein. The "mainliners" are felt to be those who are true addicts with a difficulty in contrast to those who use the oral route. Is the "mainline" a version of the umbilical circulation and the "rush" the acting-out of a primitive experience of the reception of chemical substance coming in through the placenta to the fetal circulation? This main line situation would most clearly be the nearest approximation to a return to overt womb phantasies with the idealized perceptions of warmth, comfort, and oceanic bliss that are well-known parts of the experience of naive users of opiates. The threshold of perceived drug activity changes markedly with temporary resolution of states of massive projective identification with the dosage for intended activity being much lower when partial separation has been achieved.

In each patient Dracula phantasies emerged as a transitional state between inside and outside as identification with the baby who was in the womb (coffin) in the mother (Transylvanian soil) and parasitized the woman victim (analyst mother) by direct entry of fangs into the blood supply. References to black magic included those parts of the black mass which involved the ritual eating of the placenta after the devil-possessed baby is born. These phantasies have in common a direct contact with the blood supply of the mother and come up in close approximation to material relating to intolerance to the frustration of separation from the mother. Although there are clear examples of oral sadism, I believe they represent transitional phantasies attempting to maintain a version of placental connection outside the mother's body by direct attack. These activities are all known to occur at night and seem to correlate with alarming dreams and/or states of insomnia.

According to the shorter edition of the *Oxford English Dictionary*, the word "pressure" derives both from Middle English and Old French "pressen," "presser," in several contexts:

> *I.* *Literal* and *directly connected senses.* 1. To exert a steady force against (something in context); 2. To press to death: to execute the punishment of "peine forte et dure" upon a person arraigned for a felony who stood mute and would not plead. To compress, squeeze, extract juice.
>
> II. *Figurative senses.* 1. To bear heavily on; to reduce to straits; to beset, harass. To oppress, crush. To distress, afflict. To weigh down, burden (the mind, feelings, spirits). 2. To produce a strong mental or moral impression. To urge on, compel, force.
>
> III. *Senses connected with the notion of a throng, or of pushing one's way in a throng*. I. To crowd. 2. To push or strain forward. 3. To push one's way into a person's presence, or into a place boldly, presumptuously, or insistently. 4. To venture, obtrude or intrude oneself.
>
> IV. *Combined.* Compacted or molded by pressure.

I have found these definitions illuminating in that there is a continuum suggesting different phases of the experience of birth relating to phantasies of patients who have located themselves in the birth canal experiencing a powerful mental force suggested by the above-mentioned definitions. Experiences ranging from an uncomfortable sense of pressure to torture have been frequently observed. These patients feel themselves to be victimized by a force which is out of their control and experience themselves to be passive recipients of intolerable pain which they feel as a crushing force, oppression, a torture which is frequently experienced in the transference as the violent percussive, tyrannical, violence I have previously described. Under these conditions, thinking is severely impaired as far as the capacity to develop abstract modes.

Is there a state of mind which represents the emerging active experience of an encapsulated fetal aspect of development which contains a mental process which is a primitive form of thinking? If there is a pressure-vision as hypothesized previously, the form of thinking evolving from these primitive anlage would likely be mediated through the medium of pressure. In more developed forms, pressure is related to exceeding the threshold of a sense organ, for example through hearing or vision, at which incoming sense data can be adequately discriminated. When this threshold is reached (which would be subject to individual sensitivities), there is noted a form of psychic pain. An impression is made upon the mind which impels to action. This fetal level of experience would have been developed for use in a watery environment in which threshold levels of stimulation would have to be reached by pressure as an activating principle. A patient experiencing these phenomena would likely disburden his mind of such stimuli by means of projective identification which would account for the transference phenomena which are so constant in these individuals. Is this the obtruding experience of a form of "thoughts without a thinker," in Bion's terms, which gives rise to both the phenomena of worry and the lie as a means of avoiding this painful experience of pressure?

Worry would involve those repetitive cycles of reverberating circular patterns of thought arising from primitive fetal derivation under the influence of a pressure modality. The lie in one form would involve veering off from these primitive affective experiences emerging from this fetal aspect of the mind. Psychic pain as a determinant of the inability to tolerate frustration has long been considered indefinable and mysterious, and has been intuited to be among the most important elements leading to the evolution of psychotic mental process (Bion, 1967).

In the patients I have described in this chapter, psychic pain has been the most dominant feature in the treatment and the greatest source of complaint. It is as though catastrophic feelings which seem to be imprints of the experience just before birth emerge and threaten the patient with the feeling of impending doom. The theme of death is very close in phantasy in these individuals to that of birth, and to them indistinguishable. These catastrophic expectations are mediated by a "fetal mental set," so to speak, and as they emerge, having been stimulated by sense input from the outside, there is a form of mating which occurs between the emerging fetal experience coded through pressure as an integrating medium and the incoming sense data which may not be coded for pressure if it has been integrated at a more advanced level of development. This mating of two different levels of sense experience must be subject to a set of rules which remain to be discovered. A singular feature of the mating of a fetal pressure level with an element of experience which has had exposure to the air, as it were, is psychological turbulence which contributes to psychic pain. This mating is a kind of "poor fit," a bringing together of a mismatch, and leads to concretism of thought.

If the analyst communicates in articulate speech, the patient doesn't understand, but experiences the speech as if it were meaningless sound which may be subject to fragmentation. Unless this level of experience is investigated, such interpretation of significance will be lost and the analysis will be superficial. Does understanding increase if pressure is approximated to pressure? If the tonal qualities and percussive elements of the voice are matched, there seems to be a facilitated communication, but this must be taken as a beginning speculation, the rules for which beg to be researched. Rascovsky (1960) described "fetal levels" of experience and put forward the hypothesis that these experiences were part of the emerging transference experience and would be amenable to interpretation; however, the consideration of the nature of the language utilized to communicate to the fetal level was not developed. Ploye (1973) reviewed considerations of prenatal mental life and put forward the assumption that symbol formation may well operate at levels far earlier than those usually thought to be possible, and with sufficient reason for one to be able to infer not only the nature but also the date of the reconstructed event. Dr. Ploye confined his elucidations of prenatal mental life to imprints of toxemia of pregnancy, early and late threats to pregnancy, and felt he could identify these states in dreams with anatomic precision. I have confirmed his observations and wish to extend them to the theory of thinking which evolves through the work of Klein and Bion.

In *Elements of Psychoanalysis,* Bion (1963) demonstrated a method by which a myth could be utilized as receptor for transformations of experience both in sensory and affective qualities. By segmenting the Oedipal myth into individual themes, he hinted at a structural organization which integrates a set of sensory interconnections in a coded form. This template may act as a kind of filter which links sensory representation according to a set of rules which act as a preconception, making possible a specific quality of thought. Incoming sensa would then mate with retrievable mnemic residues according to the structure of the mythic template which bears analogy to the molecular approximation of reactants at the active site of an enzyme. The mythic structure would impart a mental counterpart of stereospecificity. This is the subject of a further study.

W. R. Bion (1975) has further drawn attention in a paper delivered to the Los Angeles Psychoanalytic Society on "The Grid," to the Death of Palinurus, as an example of visual phantasy. I have quoted the relevant section of the Story from Dryden's translation of Vergil's *Aeneid* and have divided this section into eleven main elements, as the form of this story has seemed to me to be useful as a model to illuminate a series of mechanisms, including sensory phenomena, takeover by the psychotic part of the personality, projective identification, the experience of drug narcosis, demonic possession, delusion formation, and the re-entry to the mother's body representing the transformation from an air to a watery environment, each of which has been noted to exist in the material of each patient mentioned.

> Now smiling hope, with sweet vicissitude, within the hero's mind his joys renewed. He calls to raise the masts, the sheets display; the cheerful crew with diligence obey; they scud before the winds, and sail in open sea ahead of all the master pilot steers; and, as he leads, the following navy veers.
>
> The steeds of night had traveled half the sky, the drowsy rowers on their benches lie, when the soft God of sleep, with easy flight, descends, and draws behind a trail of light. Thou Palinurus art his destined prey to thee alone he takes his fatal way. Dire dreams to thee and iron sleep he bears, and lighting on thy prow, the form of Phorbas wears.
>
> Then thus the *traitor* god began his tale: "The winds, my friend inspire a pleasing gale; The ships without thy care, securely sail. Now *steal* an hour of sweet repose: and I will take the rudder and thy room supply." To whom the yawning pilot half asleep: "Me dost thou bid to trust the treacherous deep, the *harlot smiles* of race? Shall I believe the *siren south* again, and, oft betray'd not know the *monster main*? He said: his fastened hands the rudder keep, and fix'd on heaven, his eyes repel invading sleep. The God was wroth and at his temples threw a branch in Lethe dipped and drunk with stygian dew: The pilot vanquished by the power divine soon closed his swimming eyes and lay supine. Scarce were his limbs extended at their length, the God insulting with superior strength, fell heavy on him, plunged him in the sea, and, with the stern, the rudder tore away. Headlong he fell and struggling in the main, cried out for helping hands but cried in vain. The victor demon mounts, obscure in air while the ship sails on without the pilot's care."

The elements of this story, which these patients demonstrate in common, include:

1. Hope, bliss and clear weather.
2. The falling of night, descent of sleep.
3. Dire dreams.
4. The deception of Palinurus through the wiles of the traitor God.
5. Recognition of Somnus' lie and the fight.
6. Overpowering of Palinurus by Lethe and stygian dew.
7. The ocean as smiling harlot-monster.
8. Awakening before drowning.
9. The demon mounts obscure in air.
10. The ship sails on without a pilot.
11. The moral element.

In the analytic work there is evidenced a dread of the night and falling asleep because of the fear of nightmares. The ubiquitous experience of numbness and sleepy deadness ranging to mindlessness can be mimicked with a drug (stygian dew) or lethe (forgetfulness), which often involves an attempt to fight against the temptation to use a drug leading to "giving in" to the siren south, a voice like temptress promising bliss and relief from pain. The feminine nature of the smiling harlot-monster is shown by a powerful infantile maternal transference with penetration in phantasy into the mother's body giving rise to feelings of drowning, choking, in addition to painful respiratory sensations and oedema. There is always a powerful negative maternal relationship in which a dread fear of dependency upon an individual is frequently replaced by drug dependency. After the takeover phenomenon the ship does sail on without a pilot noted by disorientation in space, loss of judgment, mindlessness and loss of perception. The story above describes a movement from air to water in terms of the maternal prenatal state and may be a clearer representation of what is meant by the "death instinct."

I have made use of a variety of theoretical formulations to describe a process which can be summarized diagrammatically (see *Figure 4.1*) to demonstrate more clearly the cyclic process of transformation of phantasy elements as mentioned earlier. This diagram is by no means complete or fixed, but is rather meant to serve as a tentative atlas of mental location and to put into coherent form the series of phenomena which have been individually detailed up to this point. The designators "in," "canal," and "out," refer to discrete locations in phantasy which correspond to anatomical sites

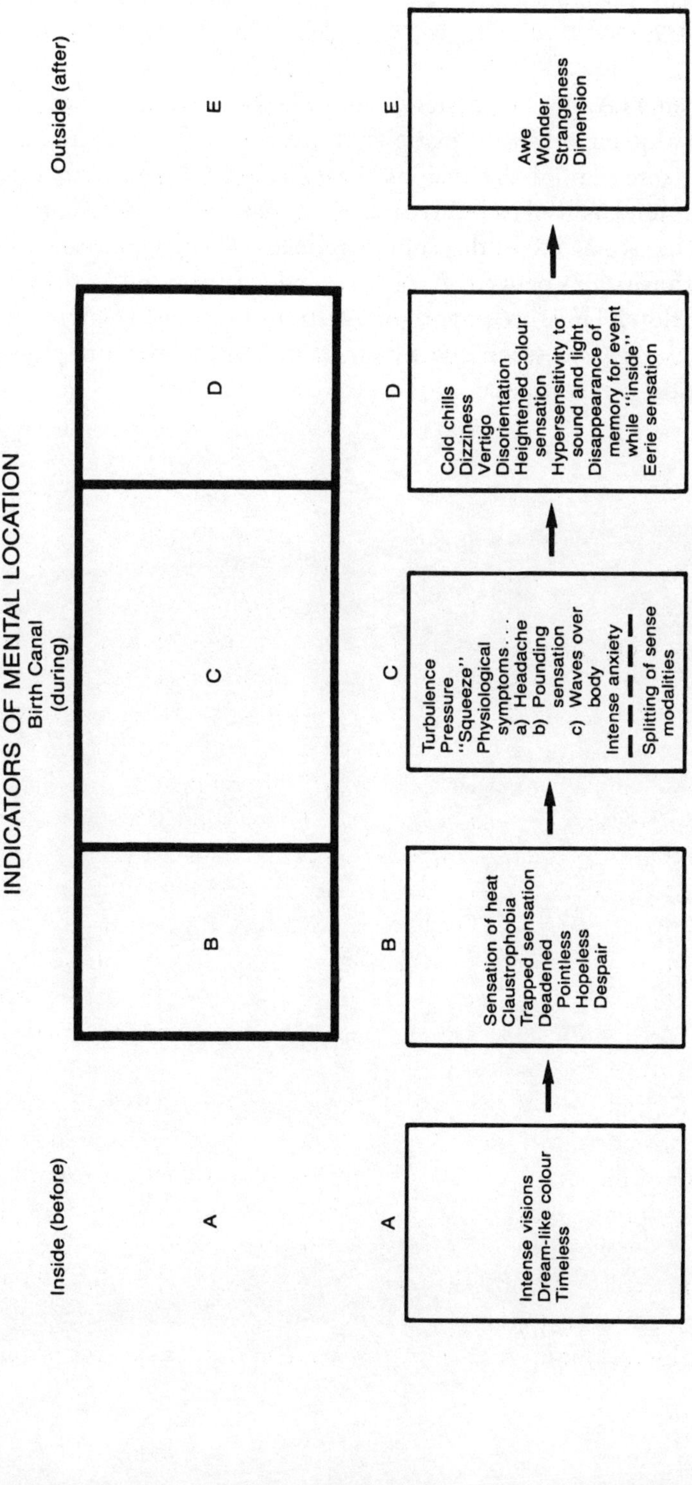
INDICATORS OF MENTAL LOCATION
Inside (before)
Birth Canal (during)
Outside (after)
A
B
C
D
E
A
Intense visions
Dream-like colour
Timeless
B
Sensation of heat
Claustrophobia
Trapped sensation
Deadened
Pointless
Hopeless
Despair
C
Turbulence
Pressure
"Squeeze"
Physiological symptoms . . .
a) Headache
b) Pounding sensation
c) Waves over body
Intense anxiety
Splitting of sense modalities
D
Cold chills
Dizziness
Vertigo
Disorientation
Heightened colour sensation
Hypersensitivity to sound and light
Disappearance of memory for event while "inside"
Eerie sensation
E
Awe
Wonder
Strangeness
Dimension

Figure 4.1

inside the uterus before instigation of the birth process, during, and after. Many of the phenomena have been detailed by other authors (Freud, 1926; Rank, 1929; Bion, 1967; Ploye, 1973; Klein, 1952; Laing, 1976; Winnicott, 1949).

The letters A, B, C . . . designate locational configurations which move through sequential transformations or remain fixed depending upon the dynamic interplay of the analytic work. These cohesive units represent states of mind as well as levels of development and serve to cohere what hitherto has seemed to be disparate experience. What are the instigators for the transformations between A, B, C . . . and what determines the direction of cyclic flow? These are important questions for psychoanalytic research in both theory and technique which affords us the awe and pleasure of exploration in the future.

Chapter 5

Primordial Development of the Penitential Transference

The prenatal anlagen of superego functioning are considered as being represented by phantasies of penitence and torture. Clinical data as to the handling of a penitential form of transference are provided as part of a process which includes obsessional states of mind. Psychic movements trigger a "mechanism" associated with the emergence of propaganda from primitive superego sources organized to stop development. This propaganda has the effect of deflecting attention from the point-on-point contact between analyst and analysand which distorts meaning and hinders reception of the interpretive process, leading to therapeutic impasse. These phenomena provide insight into a form of the negative therapeutic reaction.

Frequently in analysands who have a significant component of what often comes to be called "depression," I have noted an experience to which the patient refers as "feeling punished." This "punishment" one usually finds, has been occurring for a lifetime and often consists of a joyless, isolated experience. In this isolation, mental torture is found to exist consisting of extremely painful feeling states often associated with the presence of interruptive cruel thoughts or "voices" which lead to mental pain. These experiences come to be interpreted by the analysand as punishment for unknown crimes (Kafka, F., 1937). Pleasure or enjoyment may be dreaded even when accessible and the person lives a penitential life including phantasies of imprisonment, solitary confinement, hard labor and torture. These phantasies are frequently observed in the psychoanalytic process. Melanie Klein attributed these experiences to be harsh superego, a view with which I concur. I wish to extend the scope of this primordial conscience to having origins and profound influences prior to birth. In this way we have a marker for a distinction between the birth process itself and the birth of the character or personality.

Melanie Klein proposed on the basis of her analysis of very young children that a harsh superego is in operation before the age of three, whereas Freud believed that its formation had not begun or was barely beginning by that time. Klein (1933) points out that this superego is immeasurably harsher and more cruel than that of the older child or adult. Klein noted that in the adult the superego is by no means identical with the actual parents and is a great deal more severe than the subject's parents were in reality. She states that the younger the child is, or the deeper the mental level to which we penetrate, the more incredible and horribly fantastic the superego is. She argues that children are frightened of being devoured or cut up by menacing figures. Evil monsters like those in myths and fairy stories flourish and exert their unconscious influence in the phantasy of the child. These dreadful shapes, according to Mrs. Klein, reflect the imagined features of its mother and father and continue as unconscious phantasies into adult life. The superego of the child does not coincide with the picture presented by its real parents but is created by imaginary imagoes of them. The child's fear of real objects and its phobic anxiety is based on fear both of its unrealistic superego and of objects which are real in themselves but which are imbued with the fantastically distorted shapes of its superego (Klein, 1933).

This introjection of horrifying experiences, brought to awareness from superego sources, then in reintrojection, becomes a powerful method, by which propaganda is formed and develops as a terrifying force even though its bases are imaginary. One can see here that there need not only be the formation of harsh and terrifying images, and that these need not be the only phantasies which are reintrojected and used as propagandistic devices. Klein does not describe pleasant or seductive phantasies which are products of early introjection but concentrates for the most part on the fearsome aspects which she so clearly observed led to pathology. The very use of the word superego may be in question here as the phenomena we are describing are so different in character from the notions which Freud proposed when he described civilizing principles of fairness, moral and ethical values as versions of the parental and societal direct introjection of values. This multiplicity of "superego" phenomena implies that there are levels or many versions of "superego" which keep forming and have very different qualities one from the other.

As to the formation by the child of such fantastic images of its parents, Klein (1933) argues that the child's fears are a direct result of its aggressive tendencies. She then quotes Freud's formulation in *Beyond the Pleasure Principle*, according to which at the outset of life the instinct of aggression (death instinct) is opposed and bound by life instinct (libido).

> A fusion of the two instincts ensues, giving rise to sadism: (1) in order to escape from its own death instinct, that is aggression, the organism employs its narcissistic libido against its objects; (2) Freud considers this process as fundamental for the person's sadistic relations to his objects; (3) parallel with this deflection of the death instinct outward against objects, an intrapsychic action of defense goes on against that part of the instinct which could not be externalized; (4) the danger of being destroyed by this instinct of aggression sets up an excessive tension in the ego which is felt as anxiety so that the infant is faced at the very beginning of its development with the task of mobilizing libido against its death instinct. The ego can, however, only imperfectly fulfill this task since, owing to the fusion of the two instincts, it can no longer effect a separation between them; (5) a division takes place in the id or instinctual levels of the psyche by which one part of the instinctual impulse is directed against the other. This earliest maneuver of defense on the part of the ego constitutes the foundation of the development of the superego, whose excessive violence in this early stage would then be accounted for by the fact that it is an offshoot of very early intense destructive instincts and contains along with a certain proportion of libidinal impulses very large quantities of aggressive ones (p. 269).

Melanie Klein (1933) put forward theory explaining the unconscious sense of guilt and subsequent phantasies of punishment resulting from the activity of the aggressive instinct.

> The child perceives his anxiety as arising from his aggressive instincts as fear of an external object both because he has made that object the outward goal and because he has projected them onto it so that they seem to be initiated against himself from that quarter. He then displaces the source of his anxiety outward and turns his objects into dangerous ones. But ultimately, that danger belongs to his own aggressive instinct. For this reason, his fear of his objects will always be proportionate to the degree of his own sadistic impulses (pp. 269-270).

I include such extensive quotations so as to allow the reader to recognize clearly what has been stated before so cogently and to see clearly the phenomenological elements which will remain as invariants.

From the psychological principles of infant analysis, Melanie Klein (1929) pointed out that specific content of children's play is identical with their unconscious phantasies and that it is one of the functions of play to provide a discharge for those phantasies. Mrs. Klein showed the analogy between the means of representation used in play and in dreams and the importance of wish-fulfillment in both forms of mental activity.

Mrs. Klein (1929) further noted that in schizophrenic children, the wish to negate reality leads to the inhibition of phantasy with the resulting absence of personification. She continues:

> I have come to realize that the operation of such imagos with fantastically good and fantastically bad characteristics is a general mechanism in adults as well as children. These figures represent *intermediate stages* between the terrible menacing superego which is wholly divorced from reality and the identifications which approximate more to reality. These intermediate figures whose gradual evolution into the maternal and paternal helpers who are nearer again to reality may constantly be observed in play analyses and seem to me very instructive for our knowledge of the formation of the superego (p. 219).

Furthering her argument, she continues:

> At the outset of the Oedipus conflict and the start of its formation, the superego is a tyrannical character formed on the patterns of the pregenital states which are then in the ascendent. The future evolution of the superego towards genitality depends ultimately on whether the prevailing oral fixation has taken the form of sucking or biting. The primacy of the genital phase in relation to both sexuality and the superego requires a sufficiently strong fixation to the oral sucking stage. The imagos adopted in this early phase of ego development bear the stamp of the pregenital instinctual impulses. These early levels are responsible for the fantastic imagos which devour, cut to pieces, and overpower. The superego is made up of various identifications adopted on the different levels of development whose stamp they bear (p. 220).

Finally she concludes,

> The splitting of the superego into the primal identifications introjected at different stages of development is a mechanism analogous to and closely connected with projection. I believe these mechanisms (splitting up and projection) are a principal factor in the tendency to personification (p. 221).

An issue of primary importance is Mrs. Klein's division of the superego into evolutionary epochs, the timing of which can be studied as a function of stages of libidinal development. In her careful differentiation of the imagos of the superego in children, she has provided an important tool for designating and dating the stages in developmental difficulties in the balance of the superego, id, and ego forces. For her purposes, the superego begins at birth (Klein, 1933) and ends with the full development of the libido.

Freud's (1923) theory of the superego's formation as being a function of the impress of abandoned object cathexes is in accord with Mrs. Klein's anatomization of primitive elements within the superego as it forms. She followed Freud in providing a dynamic model for the description of the interplay of overwhelming aggressive drive (death instinct) and the means by which the violent energies of this force are modulated and structuralized by agencies of the mind (id and ego). She provides a far more primary organization of structure than does Freud, by moving back in time the functional organization of the means of taming these force utilizing Freud's original principles of ego psychology as put forward in *The Ego and the Id* (Freud, 1923).

Wilfred Bion's (1977) work of tyranny and primitive dread has ex tended and emphasized Mrs. Klein's (1923) and Freud's (1926) suggestion that birth phenomena may be implicated in the development of primitive violence. In *Bion in New York and Sao Paulo* (1980), Bion identified the beginnings of the use of imaginative conjecture in probing the mental world existing prior to birth. He sketched a loose organization depicting "mind" in the primitive stages of embryologic development and supported Freud's (1915) conjecture regarding the phylogenetic continuity of the germ plasm. A consideration of the beginnings of mind were treated both by me (Paul, 1981; see Chapter 4) and by Mancia (1981) who reviewed the literature on the development of fetal sense organization from the second month of gestation and proposed the notion of a biological clock which has the capacity for primitive temporal notation in the "mind" of the fetus.

I have used Mrs. Klein's idea of personification in which the form of phantasy taken is an index of the stage of mental development of the child and consider certain phantasies of punishment, especially penitential incarceration and torture, as having origins earlier than the immediate post-natal period as Mrs. Klein suggests. Bion (1975, 1976, personal communications) was able to intuit a fetal clock which registers maturational changes. I propose that the "clock" is triggered by primitive fetal movements and that the clock's sophistication increases with fetal growth. As the fetus grows, as Mancia theorizes, maternal and fetal physiological rhythms interface and organize the clock. Elements such as heartbeat, borborygmi, and endocrine changes help integrate temporal events in the fetal mind. Important changes include the beginning of Braxton-Hicks contractions of the uterine musculature that trigger the primitive disturbance which is connected to the experience of movement from within. We cannot know what affects the beginning of the heartbeat and awareness of the circulation bring, nor do we understand how the fetal mind experiences recapitulation of phylogenetic stages as they unfold. We can only conjecture.

What I will attempt to do here is explain a contribution to the penitential experience that occurs in both borderline, obsessional, and psychotic patients. I assume that prenatal influences, beginning with embryological shifts in development, form the basis for this complex set of mental phenomena which then become moralized, organized into mature fantasy at later stages of life, and develop the basis for harsh and extremely cruel judgements. I will also attempt to demonstrate how important communication difficulties arise as a function of this primitive "moralistic" boundary.

Here I am employing Bion's use of imaginative conjecture to propose that mental pain has its origins in the normal differentiation within the embryo as it grows and is primarily related to stimulation which the embryo and the fetus are unable to integrate. Internal movement of cell layer upon cell layer from morula through gastrula, embryo and fetus is registered but not integrated. This vast array of experience communicates with the uterine environment and the "mind" of the mother until the instigation of the process of fetal engagement and onset of labor. Then, the communication rapidly changes, effecting a barrier between the phase prior to labor and afterward. The volume and intensity of the experience of labor contribute to the overwhelming input to the fetal mind (crushing, pounding, etc.) which also cannot be contained or integrated. This forms the thrust of what Mrs. Klein called the death instinct or proto-aggressive drive and has to do with a primordial sense of overwhelming pain-to-extinction which the baby communicates in its scream to the mother postnatally. This externalization and/or projection of the death instinct-into-the-breast as Klein's formulation shows is the transformative version of object relations in their primitive postnatal state. This is what I think is meant by sadism and is what forms the beginnings of love. In this formulation, "hate" is the primitive form of love, and is a direct function of pain. Primordial pain without integration is overwhelming but is made tolerable by an affective communication link (Bion, 1962).

In this chapter I am concerned with how the individual experiences and interprets these reminiscences of primitive pain (death instinct) as punishment.

In his discussion of the Rat Man, Freud (1909) described phenomena now seen as commonplace especially in obsessional and borderline patients which take the form of a penitential transference. The patient believes he is being punished for unknown crimes and interprets psychic pain as being visited upon him by individuals with whom he is in contact, especially the analyst. The patient will often hold the analyst responsible for a distortion of what the analyst actually said. The analyst may say X and the patient responds as if he has heard the analyst say Y. The analyst's interpretation is "interpreted" by the patient, often signaled by the patient's attempt to respond by stating, "What you mean is Y." Further investigation reveals that Y is a very rapid "free association" to X (the analyst's interpretation) which the patient then attributes to the analyst. When one asks if the interpretation is remembered, one finds it is often distorted and very frequently forgotten, but the patient believes his "free association" is what the analyst has said. The avoidance of the analyst's interpretation turns out to be a means by which the patient attempts to avoid severe mental pain. The experience of mental pain may have a variety of manifestations including the rapid onset of a feeling of pressure around the head, the sudden development of an intense anxiety, or severe tension in the neck and shoulder musculature often revealed by rapid movements of the limbs, shoulders, shifts of position, and jerking movements. These muscular responses may be the patient's attempts to rid himself of extremely uncomfortable sensations which are felt to be brought about by the direct contact with the analyst's verbalizations. These behaviors typically occur when the analyst has been successful in intervening in the patient's avoiding contact. Glib, oblique, seemingly indirect ways of responding by the patient must be thoroughly intercepted and analyzed in order to allow painful responses to emerge. The patient may feel injured by very cruel, insulting voices or thoughts. He may experience being punished, or even physically slapped, and will often accuse the analyst of abusing him. This process may well go unnoticed for years in the treatment and may only emerge sadly at termination. Only when these experiences of mental pain or verbal contact with the analyst become manifest can they be sorted out. This process of misunderstanding must be distinguished from empathic error on the part of the analyst.

Freud (1909) defined obsessional ideas as transformed self-reproaches which had re-emerged from repression and had initially been related to a pleasurable sexual act in childhood. In his Rat Man case, he generalized this formulation to say that obsessional ideas can correspond to every sort of psychical act. "They can be classed as wishes, temptations, impulses, reflections, doubts, commands, or prohibitions" (pp. 221-222).

These forms of thought as interjections are what commonly replace the analyst's interpretations and are responded to by the patient's feeling injured, punished, attacked and often lead to a sensation of "pressure" either in the head or chest. This discomfort results in a feeling of need to act by immediate translation into a muscular movement or reaction. When these reactions take the form of speech, the interchange is very rapid and oblique. This process produces the feeling of bouncing off the verbalizations in such a rapid fashion as to arouse suspicion in the analyst that the verbal responses do not represent thinking in response to what has been said, but again, an oblique evasion of directly dealing with the analyst's utterance. While this form of to-and-fro communication may give the appearance of a creative free associational interchange and may *seem* to yield an understanding of the analyst's interpretations, slowing down the process of communication begins to betray the experience of the pain referred to above and is definitely *a function of velocity of communication*. As the communication slows, the patient begins to note feelings of being hurt and accused, confuses the analyst's interpretations with sarcasm from an inner voice, feels increasingly demoralized, and may comply with what he imagines the analyst wants in order to stop the pain. The patient may conversely stop all cooperation with the analyst, capitulating to a force from within which mocks, insults, derails, and threatens if the communication persists. The patient may take the part of this scathing voice from within and mock the analyst and insult him in the manner to which I have referred above. The analyst is experienced as the part of himself which is identified either as a cruel superego or victim. The successful interpretation of projective phenomena of a very primitive quality is quite essential here in order to prevent the emergence of severe feelings of persecution in both analyst and analysand. The analysis may become rapidly transformed into an experience of torture brought about by verbal interchange.

Franz Kafka's short story, *In the Penal Colony*, will serve as a vivid example of the cruelty associated with verbal communication, when the prisoner is forced to lie on a bed quite fixed by bonds while a series of sharp hypodermic needles inscribe upon his body the sentence which the condemned person is not to know until it is inscribed. An acid solution is dripped through the needles as the message from the "superiors" is inscribed; when the inscription is "understood," the condemned man is pierced through by this apparatus called a Harrow, and the "judgement" is exacted upon him. Understanding of the sentence and "enlightenment" is supposed to occur after hours of this procedure just prior to death. "Enlightenment" is supposed to bring a "beautiful peace" to the condemned and comes even to the most "dull witted." These patients, like Kafka's prisoners, experience themselves being cruelly tortured to death by "just" and "moral" sentences coming from themselves which are the interruptions to which I have referred above. Each word quite understandably evokes terror and pain and responses of stupor, numbness, sleep, and an almost endless panoply of evasion. It is therefore essential that the analyst recognize the patient's pain. Without this understanding and effective interpretation there can be no therapeutic alliance in investigating the patient's cruel transformation of interpretations which not only affect communication, but the patient's thinking itself.

As a defense against attack, the patient may refuse to speak. Any possibility of a communication being heard or noticed by this evil agency may result in such a degree of isolation that the patient may well become a fearful recluse. These patients feel that they are possessed by evil forces which observe their every move and thought and which they will take any measure to avoid. What is the nature of these inciting activities? Is there a pattern which we can observe that triggers these cruel attacks?

Mrs. X, a 50-year-old married mother of two children, notices intense sensations of quivering weakness in her legs, tightness in her throat as if she were being strangled, severe anxiety, and associated pictorial phantasies of crashes, accidents, and images of dead relatives. She also cannot stop ruminating about her imagined lapses of responsible behavior in which she feels she could have done more to prolong the life of an aged relative. She goes over every detail in severe self-reproach and is inconsolable. These associated experiences occur en bloc and are triggered each time she attempts to make "forward progress" by any means. Running errands by herself, attempts to seek work, engaging in writing, coming to her session by herself even a short walk after having driven to my office—typically result in this constellation of experiences.

Interpretations relating to separation are felt to be correct but insufficient. The quivering weakness in her legs suggests to her that she will be unable to work. She fears choking to death or becoming frightened by either the nameless anxiety or visual phantasies that she will be paralyzed and have to endure a kind of mental torture which can only be alleviated by alcohol. She becomes demoralized after these experiences and gives up for weeks at a time before she dares to venture forth again. She can regain her composure as long as someone is with her in very close proximity but will weep uncontrollably for days at a time when either her husband or children are unable to be with her. She views her life as a cruel torture and often thinks of suicide as "the only way out." She had a very brief intense vision just before sleep recently in which she saw haggard, grizzled faces of prisoners who had been in a dungeon for fifty years. She feels herself to be in solitary confinement and frequently experiences any gaps in my understanding to be evidence of my cruelty.

The failure of these experiences to remit has led to severe distrust and suspicion that I am trying to punish her. In the early period of her analysis she had complete remission of these "symptoms" as a result of psychic fusion with the analyst. As this process was interpreted, and the magical disappearance of painful experience analyzed in terms of her awareness of separateness, the persecutory ideation returned, resulting in the patient's fury, blaming me for attacking her. She terminated treatment, returning after a year during which these fantasied attacks became intolerable. She was convinced I knew about them and yet felt compelled to return to the event after consulting several other analysts who had reportedly verified my analytic credentials. Who are these persons who have obviously been jailed since her birth? She insists that the forces that terrorize her are organized to scrutinize her activities. She feels marked by the mafia for a "hit" which can only be avoided by leading a penitential life. No indulgences and constant worry are her only "cures." Penitential life is at the heart of her anhedonia.

She is terrified of the Internal Revenue Service, the FBI, even the local building inspectors. Any form of investigation is felt to be a criminal investigation whether self initiated or initiated by the analyst. All questions are felt to be prosecutorial. She is terrified lest any member of her family break the law, and even parking tickets lead to fear of arrest and subsequent torture. She had obtained temporary relief by writing conspiracy-oriented screenplays and short stories whereby she had successfully projected her internal judgmental agency into the outside world. Interpretation of this projection led to the immediate reintroduction of the symptoms for which she blamed the analyst.

Other patients with less severe afflictions who become very compliant and excessively rigid law abiders, will rebel against this name-calling attack, leading to terror by identification with the criminal, as if to say, "All right, if you're going to call me one, I'll be one!" This identification with the criminal leads to temporary relief. (One only needs to recall Max Beckmann's self-portraits to see the sinister vision of the self reflection of his personality which had been felt to have grown evil by mere witness to man's inhumanity. He has been reported to have said that he was relieved when he could see this aspect of himself.) A hypertrophied moral sense which has omnipotent proportions is a constant accompaniment in these individuals. Their imagined responsibility far exceeds possibility. Good or moral thoughts and deeds must be thought in order to stave off the bad thoughts. Conversely, obnoxious or even malevolent behavior may be felt to be compellingly necessary in order to stave off the torture. All attempts to relieve pain by the patient will involve a form of premature closure (Grotstein, 1977a), and putting a stop to communication is frequent. Acting as the condemning judge is equally frequent.

In the countertransference, I have often felt pressure to produce a rapid cure; desperate searches for the "right interpretations" and a desire to end the session or the analysis. I have wanted to accuse the patient of torturing me. I've interpreted that this is the patient's only means of having me understand what it is that he (or she) experiences constantly.

To illustrate the role of terror, miscommunication and fear of forward movement I will present in detail three sessions with a forty-year-old unnamed male who had been in analysis approximately five years. I want to present this material in as detailed a fashion as possible so as to demonstrate methods of technique which may seem unorthodox, especially as regards the necessity to interrupt the patient at key points in the session.

PATIENT: I had a dream last night that *I went to the house that I built . . . a lot of people . . . furniture and a party going on. I wouldn't call it a sex orgy, but they didn't have much clothes on . . . a lot of pillows and beds . . . an old-fashioned refrigerator. My girlfriend complained about certain design features in the house. Noise or air drafts and then that ends . . . the guys leave, and I leave and forget my clothes and come back, and meanwhile there is a formal party where others have been replaced serving hors d'oeuvres. After a while they began charging money for them which seemed unusual for a party at home, so I go home. I feel good that the comments about the home are mostly good and that there were some complaints.* I am upset that he put a badly designed refrigerator in the house, and disappointed about having sold the house too cheaply, and about not having lived in it myself. I went to look at a house yesterday. The traffic is increasing at home very rapidly. There's too much noise over the last six months. There is a great deal of heavy traffic. It's too heavily traveled. It used to be that the traffic would occur from seven to nine and four to seven, but now it's all night, and it's annoying me so I saw a house at $89,000, a piece of trash much smaller than the house I have now, and that may have triggered a lot of my feelings about the cost of houses and stuff like that.

ANALYST: You don't like drafts and noise or paying for what you're expecting to receive free. You are very disappointed especially when you discover that people do what they like, whether you feel you are in control or not, especially with respect to the refrigerator. You felt you would get a reward for building the house, and that you would go along with it. You would be in a continuous party.

PATIENT: The packaged deal, as they say. There's another issue. Am I a piece of shit or am I valuable? There have been a lot of thoughts I didn't relate. I have been looking for a cheap lot, but I changed that into not being able to afford it. I have a way of talking myself into not having money. The nice lots are $100,000; I ignore them, and I was thinking this morning, why am I forcing myself into a position of taking what's left over? This guy would subordinate until the end of construction. Why would I put myself in the corner?

ANALYST: You're still identified as the house, you feel it would be much better to be a quality house.

PATIENT: Yes. I demean myself. I took away my resources. I beat myself up. The same issue came up in the last two or three days in determining what I'll charge for consulting services. I had an interview with a man for a large consulting firm. He had a job for me, and I wanted to know what he wanted. I told him I wasn't sure. One man said he'd pay me $150 a day, so I said that was below my minimum for my level of experience, but it's really based on what I feel I'm worth and what I want.

ANALYST: Who puts the value on you? Who qualifies you? It's not the people who buy your house.

PATIENT: It seems that it's mostly me. Even if external people would call me a superstar, those people get me into a lot of difficulty.

ANALYST: This conversation seems to have a logical approach on the surface.

PATIENT: Well, what I'm hearing is, "You dumb asshole, why did you sell the house so cheap? You're a fucking fool."

ANALYST: (I then drew attention to the fact that the patient does not listen to either of us. Other factors seem to ride over, i.e., this voice that suddenly has appeared, for example.)

PATIENT: This voice is very interesting. It says, "You're going to die, you're going to die." It screams, it terrifies me. "You're going to lose your job you're going to lose your job you're going to lose your job." Then, when I sold the house, it screams, "You sold it too cheap you sold it too fast, there's nothing you're doing right," so the choice is to be terrorized or be beaten. Feels like a terrific tyrant. I hate it. (There was a break, with a sudden deadened silence.)

ANALYST: (I drew attention to the intervention between himself and myself, that something in him is behaving very much as if it does not like to be located so that it just went underground.)

PATIENT: Yes, it's like an earthworm, I remember one time when I was angry at my boss. I told him that if he'd hire a consultant for $100,000 a year he couldn't get a better one. I can know it's extremely valuable but not be sure that I believe it.

ANALYST: You seem to be off the point. You went underground, then you rode over me, so my consultantship is not valued, and as soon as you do, suddenly you don't value yourself. Yesterday you said you were concerned about wasting your time and not mine which is some indication of turning our work together into shit.

PATIENT: Which comes first, the work or my life? I have to worry about me more than I have to worry about work.

ANALYST: That's not the point.

PATIENT: I didn't really think it was, so why did I say that?

ANALYST: Yes, well it gets us off the track.

PATIENT: I don't like the feeling of being focused on at all.

ANALYST: I think you feel that there's a tyrant that maintains an overpowering, hostile scrutiny, an observer that's constantly viewing you, which is internally located and watches you so closely that it knows everything whether you're aware of it or not. It knows all your tricks and you can feel now when I focus and when we focus together that it's with that sort of eye, that sort of critical, hostile scrutiny, and then you subordinate to it and become obsequious or evade the issue.

PATIENT: Yes, I feel no choice except when I have some kind of feeling of revolt, some kind of feeling of an internal revolt. (End of session. On the following day the patient began as follows:)

PATIENT: I had a dream last night about *a room full of people, like a prison. I think it was a prison, and I'm sure they were Japanese. There was a warden who sat on a podium with a machine gun, and he wants to kill all these people, and at some point he does kill some people. Then there are still people alive, but he leaves, and he says, "I'm going to get ready to kill off the entire room," and leaves a young lady in charge with the machine gun, and she decides that's not right, so she decides she's going to kill the warden. She turns the gun sideways toward a staircase that you would have to climb. It's a very difficult angle, and she sits the gun by the door, and the prisoners know that she's going to lull the warden, but they are relieved. They are not going to be killed, but they're nervous about the rebellion. It's very clear except this woman; who is she? She is a kind of judge or a higher authority or a separate authority. There was a woman yesterday too. She might be a part of me. They are the captives, the warden and the judge, the woman. It's not the captives, but the judges that kill. The captives would not dare to kill the warden. They sit in awe and don't help to carry the machine gun.* I don't think I'm going to kill myself. I don't know, I really don't know. The dream tells me that's what I'm considering so that it's no joke that I'd carry something like that out. I don't know. It's up to the judge part. The captives don't want to. They'd be happy to have their freedom, but the judge is more serious, vindictive. She wants to kill the warden, but I don't know why. Why has the judge got it in for the warden?

Maybe the warden and the judge are like mother and father. The captives feel like the children who just want to go out and play. I feel that the warden and the judge are carrying out this big deal—you're in prison, know you're going to be set free, knowing the captives are just sitting there watching this thing go on and on. Maybe that was my view of mother and sister or mother and father.

ANALYST: And now, between you and me and the woman, I don't think you're feeling very comfortable with machine gun intercourse.

PATIENT: I used to, or I used to think I did. The warden, captives, and judge being like one person and then coming apart, and then there's just the warden and the captives, and then the warden comes apart. The warden and judge are very close, but the captives are further away. It's like a battle for custody over the children. The judge's motto is that they are going to be free if I have to kill everyone.

ANALYST: You are in conflict about what you want? Do you want to stay in for life, or do you want to crack out?

PATIENT: Both are being forced. I just want to be left alone and go play. I was thinking I should have plans for the holiday, but it has to be plans for everyday. I need plans for all of the time. That's a real problem. Last night I went to the ballet. It was superb. Someone called me. I went with her because I knew she's a drag, because I wanted to see the ballet. But there's a part of me that said that's a drag, and I have to learn how to tolerate it. She's very depressed and frightened. He's been supporting her completely—that's her husband. She's afraid that he's going to stop paying, and is thinking of schemes. What have I done? Why doesn't she love me?

ANALYST: She is felt to be an external version of what you feel on the inside. You can get rid of her, but not that aspect of yourself. There's a part of you that sees a terrified or frightened or sad or weak or ignorant or small aspect of yourself and wants to kill it. Anytime you had a sad, small feeling, there is jealousy, the warden wants to kill, where these children are the feelings which are being held hostage. Feelings are felt to be no good, they don't get free play. They're being watched like a hawk by the judge.

PATIENT: Yes. While I was watching the ballet it was very beautiful, yet I was in the presence of this depression. This girl was so depressed, and the beauty and the contrast was quite strong. I felt torn. If only someone beautiful was sitting there next to me that I wouldn't be so torn.

ANALYST: Yes, you were so depressed and frightened because of the judge and because of the state of terror in which you live.

PATIENT: Yeah, now we're getting somewhere. There's movement. It's slow. It's painful. I'm emerging. I can feel it. I am emerging, and I can actually feel it. I don't know how to explain it. I have a lot of little indications of it. I'm continuing to look for land. I continue to get up every day and figure out what I want to do. Not well, but I'm doing it. I'm seeing people and I'm working at consulting jobs with a feeling of having something to offer. It's not a strong feeling, it's a weak feeling, but it's good. I don't want to beg. I don't want to beg for a job. I have something to offer. It feels right. I'm going in a series of directions. I'm going ahead to get a real estate license. I've advertised for consulting work. I may look for land to buy and sell because it is in such demand, and I found a piece, but it may be too expensive. I'm not saying whether these will work out, but I am exploring, and it feels good to me. I think that's the modern form of telling the children to go out and play. I set up a really nice office in my home that I love. That's important but I didn't mention it.

ANALYST: I'm felt to be the judge who's not going to like it if you enjoy yourself.

PATIENT: Whose office is it, yours or mine? I must think that I took your office, otherwise I wouldn't be upset, like I don't deserve it.

ANALYST: There's the judge that you don't deserve or anything as if, in fact, there was a moral issue.

(In the next session directly before the weekend break the patient begins:)

PATIENT: There is a long weekend, and I haven't made specific plans. Yesterday I called the Sierra Club about a trip, and they said why did I wait so long, and I don't really have an answer for myself. I keep telling myself I don't take good care of myself, but that really doesn't really seem to answer it. I don't really understand.

ANALYST: No you don't, but you talk as if you do.

PATIENT: It's easy to use those words, as if they explain, but it doesn't. There's some process I don't understand very well and that I have to find things out for myself. I repeat something. I'm very good at make-believe, repeat-after-you kind of thing. But, I began to realize how much I don't know, and that's quite scary actually in a way.

ANALYST: You can repeat after me, or you can repeat after yourself, depending on who's talking, but you then have to use words like "actually" and "in a way" so that as you understand the meaning to suggest that you really mean what you say, then you erase it. "Actually in a way" is utterly meaningless verbiage, but you are reduced to that sort of talk in order to make a distinction between what you've suddenly recognized as having meaning and that which does not.

PATIENT: I'm recognizing something when I know it in my bones and when I spout things. No matter how well I theorize and all that crap, but I know how to take care of myself. The weekend is an example, but it's all the time. Ahh, we're going back to the beginning, ground zero, and I don't think I like it.

ANALYST: It sounds like you expect a nuclear attack. Apparently you're very angry about not knowing.

PATIENT: Yes, I feel that there's too much that I don't know. First there was structure, and then we ripped all of that down. The structure of not knowing is another kind of structure, but I don't know why. But not knowing is very hard for me. I just had an image of Marines working out the course, that they have to jump over a six-foot wall, reaching it and then falling down, trying again. Hitting it and falling down, like not knowing is a barrier, and you can't get through by direct assault. That's my position, and I find it difficult. But in some areas I'm able to work better than others. I run into so much trouble, and I don't know what to do. We keep coming back to that.

ANALYST: You're assuming you don't know what to do, but the part that does "know" is acting very specifically to keep from doing something. In this regard you can notice that you are propagandizing yourself here in the moment over and over by repetitive actions so as to brainwash yourself into telling you that you don't know what to do. In this regard there is a violent attack, it's felt to be a bombing attack on your capacity to live. Like the warden.

PATIENT: Those guys are all invisible. I saw them yesterday, and I see the effects of them today. That's true. I agree, and I purposely keep from doing things. The appearance is that I don't know what to do about the warden. It's like taking a ghost and putting clothes on it so that you know where it is. But that's not enough. But I don't know what is enough. Maybe I have got to know them well. I'm not sure what that means. They're going to take me over. That's the feeling that I have. If I bring them out, and making that visible, they'll take me over. I'm afraid. They've got me out now in their invisible way. But, to bring that out, it feels like they'll take me over. They'll take me over, and there's the battle. They're trying to draw me in and I'm trying to draw them out. I know that there's something going on inside of me. When I don't speak to you I feel like I'm leaving, and being drawn in. I can feel myself leaving. All kinds of activity going on in there.

ANALYST: Yes, it's felt to be much more interesting in there than being here with me. It says, "Don't pay attention, pay attention to me." You can notice the propaganda, "They'll take me over, they'll take me over."

PATIENT: Yes, it feels like a sleepy feeling that blots out my awareness. I feel lost. I feel like I'm in a maze, in a web, and I can't get free. I just had an image of a boat with a wooden cabin, a girl in it, and a tabletop. There's a battle for control of me. Who's going to have it? I don't understand who these are. I can keep fighting for control, and I don't know what the fight is. I have an image of a little baby and a woman, and she's having her cheeks rubbed. I think I want to go back to mother and be a little baby. There's another whole level of activity very definitely. Who am I? I don't know. So there's nothing left. It's like I'm sucked dry, and then I come back lifeless. The life is left behind. Maybe that's why I come back as a ghost because I leave it all in this other place. There's a lot of wooden cabinets, kitchens. Maybe I was intrigued with kitchens when I was a little boy. I wonder why the boundary is so precise. I flip from one world to the next. I do think the other is a lot more interesting. There's a lot going on there.

ANALYST: Yes, compared to your life. That might explain why there are no plans, why there is felt to be nothing going on in the real world that you feel you simply go where the action is which is inside, nowhere else. That'll keep you in, and locked in.

(The session ends.)

Many points of technique can be discussed in reference to this case which can be viewed from a variety of vantage points. Initially, I would like to draw attention to the sequential emergence of relevant themes.

1. There is a house in which some version of a "sex orgy" is occurring (his internal world) which he is recognizing that I am scrutinizing.

2. There is a powerful resistance to psychic movement and fear of change. At the same time, the drafts and noise in the house are references to inroads made by the analysis leading to a crack in the seal of the patient's isolation.

3. Identification with the container-mother-house is recognized and

directly leads to the "beating" to which the patient refers.

The beating, berating, self-reproaches are organized by "superego structures" which recognize the connection between myself and the patient and operate to get us off the track. Important in this regard is the issue of "dire foreknowledge and phantasies of prediction" which can be very elaborate in these patients. The dire warnings and fears of crashes, disasters, etc., are invoked to discourage further forward movement.

4. Devaluation of the self and what is known as narcissistic depression is the result and partially serves in the first session to distract both of us onto the issues associated with devaluation so as to avoid the further progress leading to more movements and "drafts."

5. This is a version of the phenomenon Bion (1967) has elaborated which he calls "attacks on linking" so as to engage the subject to rationalization.

6. Maintaining contact with the patient's anxiety and drawing attention to each evasion yield (with a cooperative patient) to the emergence of the awareness of the tyrannical propagandizing superego which acts to keep real contact with the analysis to a minimum. Psychic forward progress is related to direct emotional contact with the analyst under conditions in which accurate interpretation leads to the development of a working alliance which is recognized in some primitive manner. In this situation, mental location is a version of a sealed house never opened to the air. That is a primitive version of phantasies of being in the womb prior to birth. This is the penitentiary, concentration camp, penal colony which is discovered and experienced through meaningful verbal interchange. This might explain in part why meaningful talk is so hated and avoided. Bion (1967) refers to this phenomenon in his paper, "Attacks on the Linking," and points out the exceedingly important issue of psychic pain being increased with focused mental communication.

Donald Meltzer (1973) in his chapter on "Terror, Persecution, and Dread" in *Sexual States of Mind*, states, "I have come to the conclusion that intolerance of depressive anxieties alone will not produce the addictive constellation of submission to the tyrant. Where a dread of loss an addictive relation to a tyrant is found in psychic structure, the problem of terror will be found at its core as the force behind the dread and the submission". He continues, "Until such a narcissistic organization is dismantled and a rebellion against the tyranny of the bad part is mounted, progress into the threshold of the depressive position is impossible" (p. 106). I agree with Meltzer's formulation and wish to extend it by postulating the narcissistic organization is centered around maintenance of the jaillike internal world as a representation of being in the womb and of never having experienced contact with the real world. The wall or gate to which the patient makes reference in the clinical material may be more dramatically connected to the gatekeeper in Kafka's parable, "Before the Law." It is the phantasy of the uterine wall which can only be passed through by elaboration of the psychic birth process (see Chapter 4). Before the paranoid-schizoid position can develop, not to mention the threshold of the depressive position, the patient must be released from prison from which he dreads escape. He must go through the process of psychological birth. The superego structure we have traditionally recognized as the moral imperative, the agency of moral judgement, is obviously exceedingly complex. The salient point here is the gating function of the superego for the maintenance of the hermetic seal so that the patient is "protected from living and being in the real world" by propagandizing, brainwashing and censorship which threatens and terrorizes the patient. The experience of the patient's feelings are interpreted by this extremely primitive superego function, and interpretations given are verbal, i.e., "You'll choke to death, you'll be killed, don't listen to that," often given repetitively so that the patient fails to make the distinction between internal interpretations made by the "internal analyst" and the interpretations made by the external analyst. It is our job to interpret what we sense through our organs of perception. In these patients the superego reacts with foreknowledge in order to prematurely closure and stop movement in psychic space. This mental movement leads from a state of being in the womb to an "outside" state of mind. The internal interpretations act before understanding is available through true contact, and are perceived as harrowing.

7. As the analytic work stimulated the dream in the second session, the patient became aware of the nature of the difficulties. "Depression" is an inadequate diagnosis as it does not make reference to the problem of the patient never having been outside. Projective identi-

fication is also questionable here since that requires that the patient be mentally born. This state of mind, "depression," involves prebirth mnemic residues laid down in sense memories before the use of language, yet can be evoked by contact with verbal thought (Bion, 1977; see Chapter 4).

8. After considerable analytic work, the patient in the third session refers to noticing the difference between knowing something "in my bones" and "spouting things." Here he is referring to not listening to what he says until, through my intervention, he does just that and is able to make the distinction between what he means and what he has said. He must maintain enough attention, to listen to what he said, to what I have said, and retain in his mind the distinction so as to keep us on the track. If he cooperates, there will be an instigation of psychic movement which he knows will lead to pain. Thus, cooperation requires intense courage of a kind which may not be readily evident since the patient must suffer. This phenomenon is partially responsible for leading to the confusion between psychoanalysis as a penance, the psychoanalyst as a judge, jury, executioner and that process which leads to the emergence into the external world. (In my patient this involved the concrete reference to "real" estate versus the world of sealed phantasy.)

   When Meltzer (1973) states that, "factors in psychopathology such as intolerance of separation, or of depressive pain or cowardice in the face of persecution, cannot be accurately estimated" (p. 106), I would agree. In addition, meaning cannot be approximated since language has been used and even developed for the purpose of evasion. Only when the patient becomes aware of these sensitive issues of meaning which depend upon the development of focused attention can his use of language be investigated. The same qualities and capacities for attention and precise study of meaning are obviously required of the analyst if any progress is ever to be made.

9. The references to the wall in the third session are visual phantasies used as evasion, and the disappearance of contact can be traced to solid entrenchment, lifelessness, and return to the dead mental world as the session and analytic week come to a close. The emergence of visual material in which a dream-like phantasy appears alerts the analyst to a change in mental functioning which can be likened to being in a dream. This is quite a serious situation since his

dream and the world which the dream represents prevent any emergence of the contact between himself and anyone else and is used for the purpose of producing isolation in the transference.

10. The development of an effective analytic pairing must take into account the patient's use of language. I have mentioned previously the use of evasive language and increased splitting as emotional contact is approached. Demeaning and terrorizing insults are noted, especially in the second session, and are used as a further "incentive" to have nothing to do with the analyst; the attacks on linking between analyst and patient can be noted to have increasing frequency and contact. Threats and terrifying visions seem to be used by a canny agency with precise timing to propagandize and batter the patient into delinking, splitting off from contact, and attacking the capacity for hearing or paying attention to what is said. The patient will often bitterly complain of being brainwashed, sarcastically maligned, and assume that it comes from the analyst. He (or she) is often correct about the phenomena of brainwashing, and much work is necessary in order to demonstrate its origin from within the patient. As a result of having been spoken to in this manner for much of their lives at the hands of the hidden interpreter within, these people actually complain of being over-sensitive, easily hurt, and have assumed that language has little meaning except as a form of action meant either to escape or to injure. Meaning is distorted not only as a function of misunderstanding, but as a function of failure of development of language as a form of symbolic communication. Often, only technical language is trusted; abbreviations are used as if no explanation is necessary, since jargon is often not only depersonalized and general but has a standard use which is often quite concrete and free from the necessity of interpretation. The patient frequently has never experienced contact with a person who means what he says. The recognition of this by the patient often brings considerable depressive experience as there is the realization of the lack of understanding of signals. The tools for effective symbolization and thinking are often very poorly developed. In people of high "achievement" and intelligence this is isolating and may be discouraging since the increasing capacity for recognition of imitative speech and seeming thinking in themselves and others may cause a revolution in what the patient considers to be true communication. If one seems to have spoken articulate

language for a lifetime and discovers that it is merely imitative, then everything in the realm of discriminatory awareness is in doubt.

11. At this point, the analysis may became very stormy as the patient finds himself in a dilemma.

As he experiences greater contact as a consequence of marking the distinction between sincerity and oblique communication, there is increasing psychic pain. If he resists or backs off he knows it, and is subject to the painful awareness of the wasted time of his life. Each detailed analytic sortie brings him more and more in contact with the depression associated with wasted time when evasion is evidence. The analysis becomes a practical micro-environmental model for the details of his life outside. There is no more succor. The delusional inside world is suddenly invested with pain. Forays into the unfamiliar external world are fraught with shame, the recognition of extreme naivete, vulnerability, doubt, and severe anxiety. He is between the devil and the deep blue sea. The analytic work is marked by vacillations between intense hatred and delusional quasi-wakeful dream states as a means of escape. The analyst is experienced as a traitor, and no one is trusted. The analysis is maintained only under conditions of good faith built up over the years leading up to the experience. Courage on the part of both analyst and analysand is required as the mutual suffering can be quite severe. Theoretically, this stage would mark the inception of a homologue of the paranoid-schizoid position or, better stated, the schizoid-paranoid position, in Melanie Klein's terms.

12. The themes of betrayal and total mistrust become evident and are especially bitter when mixed with the mnemic residues of pressured squeezing violence, terrifying visions, flooding anxiety, dread of drowning, respiratory distress, and sudden rapid fluctuations in temperature from a sensation of freezing to suffocating heat. There is the conviction in the analysand that a medical illness is in evidence, and a hasty retreat to medical means can be a frequent result.

It may seem a fanciful model for this betrayal to consider that the sudden activation of the uterus to contraction during labor may be the traitor, once having been the peaceful sanctuary turned violent. The precipitous appearance of this theme of betrayal is an exceptionally dangerous threat to the maintenance of the analytic process and may be an important source of contribution to the negative therapeutic reaction.

At this point, extrapolating back to the conditions during labor, we can guess that overwhelming sudden bursts of epinephrine released across the placental barrier to the fetus resulted in the experience of overwhelming anxiety without the capacity for thinking transformed the experience. Does this correspond to what Bion (1962) has termed the "nameless dread"? Is this the trauma which has imprinted in nonsymbolic memory acting as a barrier, the approach to which fills the patient with terror and activates defenses against psychic movement as a reminder of the primary uterine motility during parturition? This is obviously another concrete correspondence and, although the relationship seems to configure with constancy, I think it is wise to simply note the connections without making causal inference. It is tempting, however, to accept the formulation but to do so is dangerous since it might be simply a neat explanation in symbolic terms for an experience which cannot be truly remembered in symbolic terms as we know them.

The signal experiences forming the so-called superego sources then alert the fetal organization to impending extinction. Thus, the flooding of primitive nonsymbolic mnemic residues serve to halt psychic activity in response to these emergent feelings. The analysand feels the analyst is trying to kill him, and suicide/ homicide seems to be the primary emotional experience in the transference. Not until the patient becomes aware of the patterning of the waxing and waning periodic intensity of these experiences is he able to believe both that be will not die from these feelings and that the tyranny of the internal propagandist has been organized to "save" the subject from certain death. The organization developed as "protection" becomes the "jamming" interruption which stops experience. Only with the courage and patience required to maintain the treatment do the experiences of primitive undifferentiated hatred and love begin to emerge for analytic sorting. This then requires the intense cooperation of the patient in order to be able to "contain" the experience of these violent proto-emotions and to think them through. This process must be literally worked through time and time again with the permutations and combinations which present themselves in mixed fashion. With the successful emergence of these primitive feelings of love and hate, sexual sensations make their entry, often perceived as confusing and inappropriate to the circumstances, and may be severely criticized and/or shut down by the moralistically cruel "superego" formations. Thus these feelings may be secondarily treated as shameful by the internal interpretive agency. Here, life can be seen to be interpreted as death and vice versa if we consider the emergence of feelings as a paradigm for life itself. Can this be the origin or anlage of reversal or reaction formation which Freud voices in relation to obsessional neurosis?

13. The question arises as to the distinction between superego perverse origins as a function of envy versus those arising as a function of prenatal influence. The problem seems to be preverbal traces coming through in reflections of uterine rhythmic "contractions" having to do with the percussive repetitive sound which has a blocking action to thinking. The repetition of percussive sound has an unpleasant effect on the ear of the listener including the speaker and eventually functions to put a stop to listening in the speaker. This particular phenomenon is not only a function of a prenatal experience; however, it is more weighted toward that experience. Envy involves a spoiling attack and devaluation but lacks the sense of *pressure* and repetitive percussiveness. The phantasies associated with the walls being impenetrable and breaking out as a fear seem specific to the prenatal transference. In addition, phantasies of flooding, drowning and the comfort of being locked in with the dread associated with the awareness of forward movement have not in my experience borne reference to envy which needs for its development *a recognition of twoness* and an awareness of a gap between the self and other. In this reference to superego, I am referring not to the mature agency of judgement but only to reactivity evidenced by recognition (scrutiny) *of a change* followed by a means *of stopping* the change. This is as on-off mechanism, to use a mechanical analogy, and not a process which involves weighing evidence, thinking, concern or more developed processes. Perhaps the use of the term superego may be confusing here because of its more developed qualities than used previously in psychoanalytic theory. However, this primordial function has considerable importance because it does function as a primitive form of judgement so that the information which would have been gathered by an agency of mature judgement cannot be taken in and always results in precocity and premature closure.

This is not to say that what is classically known as the superego does not develop and operate. But because of the power of this primitive stopping mechanism which is related to phantasies of death and fear of impending disaster (if one is born, one dies), this powerful mechanism takes precedence over more developed processes of judgement and functions as a Draconian conscience. Therefore, all forward progress leads to dread at least one source of which is propagandizing, repetitive signalling mentioned earlier. This is certainly more primitive than the Talionic revengeful treatment-in-kind form of conscience which has at some base a link to fairness.

To summarize, repetitive percussiveness recognizable in tonal elements, pressure, phantasies of drowning, being locked in and flooding, a rapid attack on forward movement and Draconian elements of judgement are some of the distinguishing factors between the "envious superego" and the developmental elements of superego sources having their origin in prenatal development.

14. The analytic work suddenly takes the form *of instrument building,* setting up new directional means for the analysand to understand the meaning of his newly found emotional stages. Now, feelings which had been kept in mental coventry in varying degrees of differentiation arise to awareness and require the analysand's reintegration from a new vertex. In this way there is an increasing richness and meaning to mental life. The analysand then has the problems which are associated with new input to awareness which have to do with selectivity and sorting. It has been my purpose to only briefly sketch this out now, as I believe this topic deserves to be treated separately.

Chapter 6

Studies on the Phenomenology of Mental Pressure

A series of psychoanalytically referent phenomena identifiable in the transference are presented which relate to a hypothetical series of coordinates in mental space. These coordinates are markers of the transitional states of mind which relate the prenatal mental world to the postnatal and vice versa. The relation to pressure, mental movement and greed are explored as junctions of the prenatal transference. The boundary between pressure and fully experienced thinking and feeling is explored as a function of threshold. The phenomenology of pressure states are sketched to elucidate control mechanisms which have functions in stopping or braking mental functioning. Mood states related to mania and depression are also related to the regulation of mental pressure.

I have been enjoined by my intellectual forebears to attempt to discover a set of coordinates by which to demonstrate navigation points in mental space. Not only to find a path within the mental realm by which to develop a personal course, but in a larger sense to venture into the world of Virgil and Dante, Blake and Milton, and to mark the boundaries of those mental spaces which can be located by such cartography. You will say, and rightly so, that is a Promethean task beyond the modesty which is appropriate to the scientific explorer. Perhaps this is the overbearing megalomania of the undisciplined, all of which must be considered. However, the problem dictated by the vectors up and beyond or below and downward are not simply solved by a blind appeal to metaphor. These are denotative statements of direction which have a continuity in the history of at least Western poetry and religion and have been represented by detailed structures variously as Elyseum or heaven/Hades or hell. All this will be familiar to the reader and there may be question as to why bother now with what seems to be so self-evident.

All my work as a psychoanalyst, the tools made available by seemingly simple matters of "direction" brought to bear by Bion (1965) have made a fundamental distinction without which I would be crucially compromised. To state the distinction basically, does the person with whom one is in connection move toward or away from you? In no way has there been physical movement, so in what sense do we note a way toward? Do we merely accept the manifest mental behavior represented by verbal thought and base our assessment on content? Are we able to actually perceive the mental appearance and hence disappearance of an individual from the "contact-in-the-field between," which we come to recognize as the *sine qua non* of real growth. As usual in the mental realm one is defining a process which is beyond "sense" but borrows from sense in a way that there is something which refers to contact (a tactile word) but which cannot be apprehended by the organs of touch. Nonetheless, I will have to rely on the reader's experience of knowing what it means to feel oneself to be in emotional contact with another or not.

These introductory remarks seem to me to be necessary in order to render the context in which they are perceived meaningful and thus extend the nature of the importance of mental coordinates. Toward and away, then, as primitive vectors are observable in the operations involving presence and absence and those manipulations of the psychic field which are signals of emotional or mental pain. This phenomenon of mental pain seems to be a quality which is ubiquitous in human nature and which when noted by the individual consciously or not, often eventuates in a change in direction, usually away, from the stimulus inducing the experience of pain. In the psychoanalytic process there can be quite a body of information about where the analysand travels mentally when he or she leaves what would be perceived as a point-on-point presence and what he or she and the analyst might find in that location.

Melanie Klein (1946) and her colleagues have detailed some of the phenomena associated with this "disappearance" or mental absence while in the presence of another and have discussed a being-inside or a powerful omnipotent fantasy of entering into the insides of the analyst as a transference object standing for the mother. This in and outness, then, can correlate with presence and absence, appearance and disappearance and has markers to which I have referred in an atlas of movement of psychic space (Paul, 1981; see Chapter 4). This movement specifically involves a phantasy of either being-in-the-womb without having been psychologically born or in a more mobile state of in and outness in reference to the capacity to tolerate mental pain. It is in relation to this background that I wish to continue my elucidation of the general process I have observed in many individuals treated over 15 years. This process will involve the beginning denotation of the set of coordinates surrounding the in and outness which has been variously named projective identification, being-in-the-womb, mental retreat, and so on. These coordinates correspond to a gateway to states of mind which have their origin in the prenatal world and are coded in our external world in moral terms.

In order to further develop this theme, I need to introduce the concept (and experience) of mental pressure which is a boundary phenomenon and of enormous importance to the understanding and charting of these inside-outside states of mind. Even though I must rely on my own experience of feeling, I must say that I can experience the "sense of pressure" from these individuals and find that my experience which often is apprehended without words can be verified by the analysand through my interpretations of what has been transmitted to me. I have taken as verification for the experience of pressure something similar to the following. "I think you are experiencing what I would call a sensation of pressure." (Yes, they would agree.) "I am noting an unpleasant pressure sensation on my face and upper arms, and I have trouble opening my eyes. It feels as if there is a force pushing on my face." This sensation can then give way to either: (1) a deeper retreat and darkness and even a sense of quietude and relief attended by the awareness of mental absence in the transference, following the pressure if the direction is away and in; or (2) by an intense sensitivity to light and sound and a sudden sensation of chill if the direction is out and toward. This latter experience is usually attended by psychic pain and forms an in-out axis which has been referred to as projective identification. It must be differentiated from the states of mind in which parts-of-the-self are split off with a corresponding sense of loss or absence of mind in the patient. The in-out axis is a more total geographic projective identification in Meltzer's (1967) terms and may represent stages of the memory of the birth process. I wish to detail the observations about this state of pressure further as there is a profound experience of augmentation and/or diminution of this pressure in the transference.

The following figure represents a considerable synthesis which I will explain. The minus sign stands for the inside state which is graduated into stages associated with mental movement or emergence. The letters A, B, C and D represent discrete stages of experience which I have described before. (See *Figure 6.1.*)

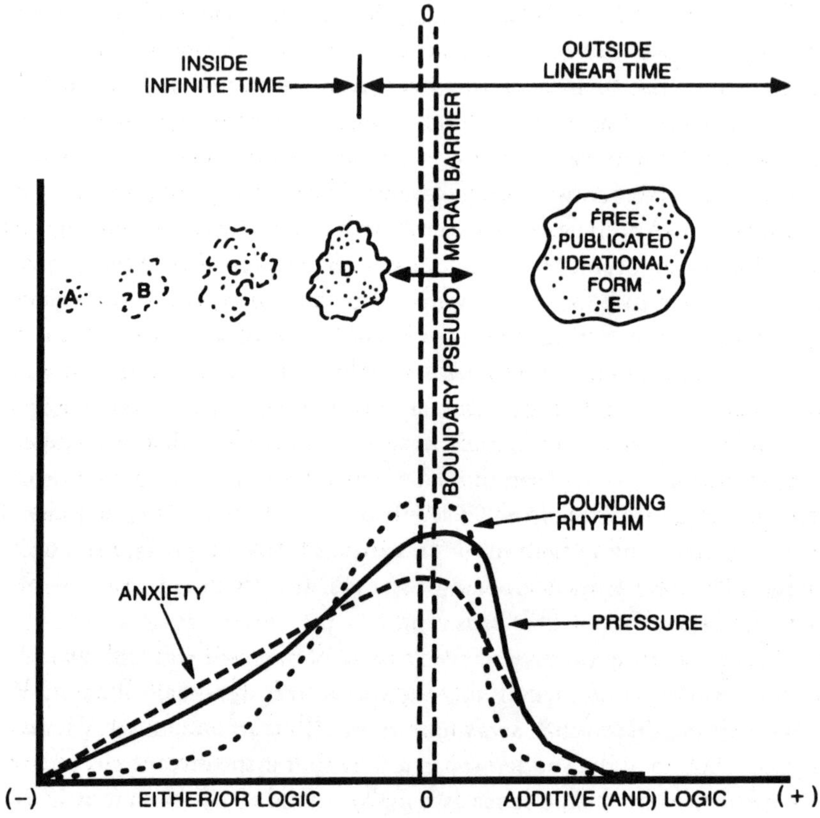

Figure 6.1

These stages are sequential and associated with progress in a session or sessions in the analytic work over time. Each letter represents a state of mind. There can be movement in both directions, A through E or the reverse. The states of mind include groups of experiences which I have noted to be constantly conjoined. The further toward the left side of the diagram, the lower is the pressure and with the approach to the zero coordinate (the precise juncture between in and out), there is an increasing intensity of pressure, dread, severe anxiety, violent fantasies and fear of acting on them. There is also a rhythmic beating quality which maximizes and then releases, dropping off considerably once inside. In the inside states of mind, there is no "and" logic, only an "or" conjunction possible hence the experience is one track. On the inside, time is infinite, changing to real linear time as one reaches zero coordinate and passes to the opposite (right) side.

This is a very skeletal description, yet contains the essence of many thousands of observations and has held its form thus far in my experience. As one can see as the individual moves from state of mind A through E, there is a considerable degree of mental pain which crescendos step by step with increasing terror and desperate attempts to stop or derail the progress. There is in the transference an experience of the painful phenomena present in both members of the pair. "Interpretations" given by the patient suggest impending doom, catastrophe and death with an intensity close to panic fear. The experience is felt as punishment and interpreted thus. These experiences have considerable significance in that they are subject to definitive "pseudomoral" interpretations by the individual undergoing the experience and are part of the process of evolution of an idea from imaginative conjecture to rational conjecture to publication. These "danger" interpretations serve to stop the development and hinder or completely stop the emergence from one state of mind to another or from one stage of an idea to another. This is an important form of derailment used to "save" the individual from danger and is a function of a mental obstruction of a relatively primitive state of mind.

There is a misapprehension as a result of mentally transforming a phenomenon by means of a moral judgmental tool. The result is a pseudomoral approach, a designation of badness which is essentially obstructive. There is a failure to understand the phenomena in question and the experience under transformation is not perceived or preserved. Hence, there is a loss of meaning because the experiential phenomena are reduced to simple categories, good or bad, not good for what or bad for what. There is subsequently an overuse or predilection for primitive conscience mechanisms acting as a primary brake on experience. Judgment then becomes misjudgment or a perversion of accuracy under these conditions. When there is powerful pressure emerging, there is moralized power turned against the pressure. Might is right in the sociopolitical context as a countervailing force to pressure. Then whatever can stand up against the pressure is designated "right" by the experience of mental pain. This pseudomoral form of "interpretation" can be found to mark the boundary from in to out or from out to in. The shift from phenomenologic experience to pseudomoral interpretation then is an important signifier of the zero coordinate allowing a kind of "navigational fix" in psychic space. If the interpretation given to the self by the conscience is pseudomoral, this evokes an obstruction stopping the movement and puts a stop to linking. Whatever is perceived by oneself, then, is "bad" under these conditions and all discovery or self-revelation is analyzed under the force of pseudomoral dictates. The obstruction and self hatred resulting produces a rapidly developing depressed state of mind. The story of the oppression of the Jews in Egypt and the myth of dividing the waters to allow passage is a kind of model for the release from this penitential state of mind. Let my people go is the injunction which desperately cries out for freedom from oppression. This penitential trap is certainly as common an institution in the external world as it is in the internal world.

Thus far there has been a designation of inner and outer, dark and light, cold and warm, pressure and its absence, trapped and free, flat and three-dimensional, timeless and adherent to an awareness of linear time as a series of clinical phenomena which can be used as markers of the boundaries I have previously described. I have deliberately focused on the elements of the birth experience as they have been the first to have been clearly observed and also provide a kind of grounding for the extension into the darker realm, the visceral darkness of the prenatal world. I was sure to make observations not only of the mental world immediately antecedent to the onset of labor but also to focus on the developmental elements in a much less systemized manner as the observations are fewer and I have less experience of them.

The approach to this underworld becomes a matter of forming a sketch and I have been impressed by the consistency and repeatability of a realm which becomes the repository of the beggars, liars, prisoners, torturers, the dumbstruck, the intelligent and stupid, the dunces who only repeat and can never learn from experience. Not simply the murderers, but the torturers and the victims, the legacy of a life experience called inhuman, but in a conceited way we could say protohuman. How scientific! Does the cat playing with the bird or mouse realize he is being cruel? Does the child eat when he realizes he is cruel to his food? This is considerable freight for the educated man to bear. How does he go into this world with his bag of woes? We are now below the surface, swimming in Freud's supposed-to-have been, primarily repressed world, and by this time there will be a considerable turbulence being set up in the mind of the listener or reader. To the rescue we have an ancient evolutionary trick. Put the skeleton on the outside and make a carapace out of it. Like hermit crabs, we venture scuttling from place to place, fending off predators or we hope—assuming protective coloration. The "as-if" defense and set of mechanisms is an inheritor of an ancient survival mechanism of forestalling extinction. The "borderline" is not simply another excuse for calling names, but represents a thin barrier between the Freudian-Kleinian unconscious and that which extends into the genic inheritance. Why is it so impossible to assume that there is a mental counterpart to the body chemical translation of experience? Do the states of mind from the invertebrata enter into the pseudo-vertebrate adult world? It is only an illusion that we see adults out there—the plethora of states of mind which can dominate are staggering. The theme of the armored creature to me has vast significance in the modern world as never have the forces been so definitively final and so profuse. Why then, in language and being should there not be the greatest dissimulation, protective coloration and resistance to being eaten or destroyed?

The vertebrate world is a very small area of this domain. There are profound changes in state of mind when the vertebrate state is reached. Being able to stand-on-your-own is a major accomplishment. This is separate and distinct from dependence. One can never avoid intense dependency, but that is separate from self-reliance and an architectural or structural ability to get around the place on one's own.

The invertebrate experience awes one's temporal senses. There is something repellent about relating us to the "spineless" as is the effective primitive verbal transformation into pseudo morality. Spineless, however, can be descriptive. One can see that today that descriptiveness in this context may only be used that way by paleontologists. Freud suggested archaeology as a model for the psychoanalytic process, but perhaps we will have to go further if we increase our time scale beyond the civilized. It is the cloak of civilized behavior that we can see without the capacity for concern, without the linkage between feeling and thought, without the deep capacity for passion other than blind hatred that we call borderline. But what happens when this is not only a psychoanalytic or psychiatric exercise in horticultural rarity? What is it that fills our society with so many of these exoskeletal invertebrates that the world has changed drastically and perhaps forever in the past 40 years?

That question can only be guessed at by the theory that the mothering has been inferior, or have the terrors become more powerful, has the rate of development been so rapid that the integrative process is saturated by too much, too fast, has there been an increasing identification with the mechanical, is there less time to digest? All must be involved and is beyond my purpose to develop the causal links if there be any. Nonetheless, these amalgamated, part mechanical, exoskeletal invertebrate forms exist indicating a kind of fragility never before noted on a general level. Can we say in general that the capacity for toleration of mental pain is decreased, or has it always been thus? Certainly in our work we see this in our consulting rooms with considerable frequency.

Three men in their early to late forties came for consultation within two weeks. One was a highly successful scientist, another a skilled chief executive of a major corporation, and a third an academic physician. All were convinced they were fraudulent, that they could not actually think, they said, and that they had experienced abject depression which they kept to themselves for years. They noted a severe blunting of affect and felt there was a huge wall between themselves and the world. They noted painful dreams in which all three reported strong images of monsters and when one inquired as to their nature, all three put their hands above their heads motioning with them to outline the shape of a large-headed form which curved and tapered to the end. They were frightened of these images which were responsible for two of these men seeking consultation.

On further examination, there were hostile voices or thoughts generating a discouraging, indeed despair-inducing running dialogue.

Remarks were made sarcastically with finality and absolute certainty, cruel remarks that could be gradually separated into what the patient thought was true and what was not. This is an essential clinical point, the one asked if the patient thinks that statement in question was true or not will often with relief note that they do not think it is. Then, the careful sorting of what is propaganda and what is felt to be accurate gives the patient an actual process which they can begin to do more and more with on their own, especially as a result of their noting that these cruel and viciously critical voices continue beyond the confines of the session. Further trigger phenomena can be found and associated which demonstrate aspects of the use of these "critical phenomena" as control mechanisms (Paul, 1989; see Chapter 5). The analytic working pair now becomes a highly relevant and practical part of the perceived essential aspect of regular life. Not as a distortion produced by the analysis; that is an induced illness, but as a means to reduce confusion and mental pain. For example, if the patient is being called stupid, unable to think and fraudulent repetitively, and he can be aware that his work has proven accurate, is respected and that these odious accusations are false, then he discovers that his feelings have been induced by the indiscriminate belief in these unexamined streams of obloquy.

The continued experience of these hostile voices when heard may lead to the awareness of the increase in the sense of pressure immediately felt by the analysand. The analyst can notice in the field between a sense of anesthesia or benumbing sensations which can either be quite physical or less powerfully may be virtually mental.

This sense of pressure, although at least extremely unpleasant and usually mentally painful, is a frequent quality which can be seen in many patients and often in everyday life. Indeed there can be an "addiction" to pressure so that processes associated with initiation of action and motivation especially in relation to decision-making are dependent on the individuals generating the experience of pressure to be able to "function."

In the addiction to pressure, one "fills" with pressure, usually "self-evoked" by internal methods, or by selection from outside sources. This is done when the pressure is "off." There is a strong tendency to maintain the continuity of pressure, often in order to maintain capacity to "function" where "functioning" involves the maintenance of the performance of a task which often can be highly demanding. There can also be a kind of pressure for pressure's sake.

Pressure may be used as the organizing force of "productivity." As one 40-year-old professional man stated,

> When pressure is the stimulus, there are several features of the experience which are consistently linked within the context of a life organizing pattern. There is no enjoyment, the primary goal is to get the job done and hence the experience over with. This experience can be education, "recreation," personal relations, work, etc. One can immediately see that huge categories of life experience are included. Motivation often comes from the intent to win. The mental pain associated with the use of pressure then leads to an addition pathomnemonic category, procrastination, and the final end or goal is to relieve the pressure once started with.

A 50-year-old attorney stated that he felt that pressure was utilized until it created pain.

> Then one increases the pressure to increase the anesthesia. The additional pressure then carries me to deadness and numbness. Then one continues whatever experience one started, now no longer feeling the pain associated with overload, which then leads to explosion.

The "cure" to the dissatisfaction and dysphoria produced by the pressure-anesthesia cycle is to do more and more, or to take in more and more. More and more eventually deadens further. One then must back up to the point antecedent to the pressure leading to pain.

> "When I am feeling less pressure," the 50-year-old attorney continued, "I do not know whether I am really feeling less pressure, or am I selling

myself a bill of goods? Then I do build up pressure to other conditions. A typical goal is the creation of an 'income stream' that does not have to pay on an hourly basis—the passive income which becomes the goal of making money while you sleep."

A typical phrase that this patient, and others like him, frequently use is "up to a point." There is a quantitation of experience in which the feeling becomes anesthetized. Once one has gone past the "point" one loses control. Then one must step up the pressure to deaden the pain associated with being out of control. That is when extension often occurs. One increases the "space" by adding a new experience. This relieves the temporary pressure by changing the venue and increasing the space.

In finance, this frequently means overextension—undercapitalization, often mistaken for greed, which is deliberate. Greed can be a matter of terminology. Here, I wish to distinguish greed from its moral connotation and note its presence as another constantly conjoined element in this personalitycharacter structure. There may be involved:

1. Inadequate containment by early parental experiences, including the prenatal world, such as maternal toxemia, diabetes; and other forms of severe illness in the maternal environment, translating to the fetus and infant.

2. There may not be an effectively introjected series of good objects leading to severe psychic pain and lack of regulatory ability to relate to the immaturity of the nervous system. There is poor regulation of input or intake in which the volume of experiences can be adequately processed for the level of development. When the experience taken in cannot be processed through feeling and/or thought it often becomes a "bolus of experience"; a beta element, unable to become alpha (Bion, 1962), which cannot be organized through a constructive transformative language.

At this level of experience we have a blurring of distinction of thought and feeling. We do not have a language for describing the distinction, but there is more or less a distinction. We know that one route is somatic/sensory (more neural, less mentalized) and can lead to certain phenomena known under the rubric of psychosomatic illness. Processing sensa in a sophisticated manner, such as in "sublimation," requires a neutralized, energy which forms a mental language, enabling thinking and essential for learning and knowledge transmission.

This is a key distinction between learning from experience and continuous growth, and the failure to be able to utilize the information or experience and transform it into a wisdom which can be passed on. The mental language may only be usable for elaborating connections, and is usable in a scientific context, bringing observations together and making connections (Bion, 1962).

Excitation is not equated with feeling. Excitation leads to anxiety, which leads to pressure. A frequent condition which can be observed in patients that are dominated by the sense of pressure is what is called stress. Another typical symptom of overwhelming stress and "burnout" is a kind of insomnia in which there is early morning awakening and counting. The question is will "the problem" get "counted out" and resolved on a course of action? Note the passive voice in this context.

In the thought cycle, the input utilizes numbers, such as economic figures and the output serves as an excess of energy to neutralize it. That is the act of putting one to sleep. The output happens to be plans, conclusions, directions of a strategic nature, i.e., buy this . . . sell that . . . develop income stream . . . cut expenses . . . pay debts. . . these orders get fed back into the system which serves as a direction for the new day's functioning. . . "I must do this and this and this." Now the system is on overload with a continuous repetition of the cycle. The cycle become a method of "handling" feelings. Thus we have feelings, and/or anxieties that are the result of overstimulation being transformed into orders or directions.

One sees, then, that the output of plans and directions fuels the next action, which is obligatory, or seems obligatory, and leads to continuous mounting pressure. For example, initially, one sets the goal to do something 100 hours per month; second, the next question is, how can one improve once that goal is reached to 120 hours per month, which is then fed back to the cycle utilizing the product as orders leading to pressure. The pressure leads to anxiety, which then progresses to anger and frustration, further to resentment, rage and hatred. One is then dominated by that series of feelings which excludes poignancy, love, tenderness, or gentleness. In order to change the system, one must stop using the effluent as the driving mechanism, or the driver. One, too, must tolerate feelings emerging . . . uncertainty and anxiety as a result of moving in a different direction, that is, not selecting the one that, say, takes the product, i.e., the increased result having been met, and then feeds it back as a set of orders.

Another example of a transformation of pressure includes a state in which a 33-year-old male businessman found himself living inside his object in a trapped state. He found that, somehow, he would experience enormous pressure which would be relieved by the visual fantasy of being rectally penetrated. At that moment, he experienced a relief of pressure and the pain was actually denoted in the sessions by his hands being squeezed under the sides of his head. He found it very difficult to pay attention as a result of his preoccupation with an internal voice which said, "I am caught between what you are saying and the interpreter, I do not know how to disregard the internal voice." I am bored, a voice says "go bang your head against the wall," which is a replaying repetition leading to autohypnosis, distraction, moving on the point, and a full stop off-track. I was able to notice that thinking, however, led to mental contact, a sense of motion, which then was perceived as on-point. Subsequently, there is the experience of intensified enormous pressure and severe anxiety as a function of being on-track. On-point, then, can be recognized as associated with the experience of pressure. "That pressure is an experience felt physically on both sides of my head, as if it were being squeezed from the outside in. As if there were hands, or something painfully pushing on it." One can then see that there are issues of sexualization of pressure and issues that involve one's orientation in mental space related to pressure.

A 30-year-old male writer had a dream of being sexually penetrated by someone while others were watching. This was perceived and associated to as the sexualization of jealousy and pain. The pressure was related to deadlines, having to do with a writing assignment. The fantasy of being penetrated, again, removed the pressure and established a sexual purpose. There was a setup of the phantasy of the primitive conscience on the outside, either in the analyst, or elsewhere. That essentially was the cure for the pressure.

> "Why do I set this up now," he said, "this pressure? A break is coming up. I load myself down and then I have the idea that I can get it all done, and then I have a feeling of relief, so I push to get it all off. One, I set the order, first X, then Y. Two, I then try to carry out the order, which is associated with relief. And three, I must have thought that all the anxiety associated with loss would go away by the establishment of tasks and the induction of pressure."

Another patient, a 40-year-old professional, regulates pressure through the use of imagery.

> The use of imagery establishes distance as a means to diminish the sense of pressure. In this point, there is a particularly difficult set of problems. When the sense of pressure is gone, I feel lost. When the sense of pressure is up, or high, then there is no desire. So, the problem that I have is orientation without pressure. I have to have pressure in order to feel any orientation. Then I end up visually distancing because the pressure gets so big, so great, that I cannot tolerate it and then I feel lost. The lost state involves having lost the place in mental space and the previous topic that I was involved in is lost. So, it is either disorientation without pressure, then adding pressure resulting in having to distance from it which then leads to disorientation again as a consequence of being lost.

Pressure, as previously noted, substitutes for the category of feeling states we are accustomed to associating within object relations on the outside . . . that is, postnatal states in which there is a field of feeling between the mother and the baby that mediates the experience of an emotional link through air (gaseous) medium rather than water or a liquid medium. The latter state is associated with the tendency to experience pressure and the pressure serves to substitute for primitive affective experiences rather than those associated with either paranoid-schizoid states or depressive states.

Although this may seem far too simple a distinction, it is useful as a means of describing a derivative of the prenatal state associated with change and labor.

Observations recently from Piontelli have added to Bion's psychoanalytic extensions of Freud's and Klein's conjectures in relation to the birth experience. Alessandra Piontelli has observed fetuses and described their behavior in utero (Piontelli, 1987). She has differentiated early states of "behavior" from states just prior to birth, such as sucking, breathing movements, and "manipulation of the cord," in her cluster of observations during fetal ultrasonography Piontelli (1987).

I have concentrated on superego formation anlage as a function of the pressure transformations of the prenatal states; massive onset of pressure prior to birth, and the medium of sensory experience being transformed through a watery medium which utilizes pressure as a means of transduction of an impulse from the outside world to the inside, or the inside to the outside (Paul, 1981; see Chapter 4).

Piontelli has observed qualities in-the-womb which are sensuous (interpreted by induction) and withdrawn, character types which she feels extend to their expression clearly in postnatal development These behaviors are demonstrated in a two-year-old psychotic girl, whose difficulties are shown to date to her prenatal life and traumatic birth. Piontelli's patient relives her past life, providing her with an intense, seemingly endless sensuous pleasure protecting her from feelings of intense jealousy of a very primitive kind and from having to reexperience her traumatic birth (Piontelli, 1988). Donald Meltzer (1975) has described similar cases in autistic states and emphasizes both the intensely sensuous qualities and the overwhelming possessive jealousy that these children have. I believe that these cases represent a spectrum and that the case of Piontelli happens to be extraordinarily clear, as is the case that I presented in Chapter 4. Piontelli's findings are clearly reproduced in cases that I have treated in the last 15 years during the psychoanalysis of adults.

I have previously described phenomenology in relation to the stages of psychological birth, and the states of mind which exist as vestiges of that state, into adult life previously (Paul, 1981; see Chapter 4). Ther is extension of that work into the phenomenology of the penitential transference, which has a clear basis in prenatal life and is associated with memories of traumatic birth.

What has become apparent to me is the extent to which derivatives of this prenatal state, with or without traumatic birth, become evidenced in the psychoanalytical sessions in cases which would have been diagnosed narcissistic to borderline, including the spectrum of obsessional qualities. I believe that this is of major significance to both manic-depressive illness and borderline-narcissistic disorders. I will develop an hypothesis as to the relation in manic-depressive disorders linked to what has been a switch process, by W. E. Bunney (1971). The earlier observations, in the early and middle 1960s, involve 24-hour cyclic manic-depressives who switched from mania to depression and back again with clock-work regularity, and who were used to lend evidence and meaning to the catecholamine theory of mood. Many different correlative metabolic observations were made during those years, later and even into the present trying to establish a chemical trigger which could evoke the switch from depression to mania. These observations involve numbers of the catecholamine groups, the 17 hydroxysteroid derivatives, cyclic adenosine monophosphate and the indolamines.

One could never make clear whether the correlative changes of these various compounds with behavioral change were primary or secondary. The time constants of the most sensitive compounds to sharply change in any measurable way were matters of hours and days, and yet it is obvious that our moods change in milliseconds on the basis of a single thought or external experience. Nonetheless, one is left with the reality of those observations, which continue to be made, especially of the sudden switch from mania to depression and vice versa. What we must differentiate, now, instead of states of chemical composition of brain, which do not yet have the resolving power to demonstrate with clarity, are states of mind which do correspond to the time constants mentioned before.

The Induction of Mental Pressure

Pressure, and the change from intense pressure to diminished pressure as one form of experience linked with its opposite low to high pressure, are, to me, key elements which are associated with time change from mania to depression. Curiously, these states of change of "pressure" define the shift between the "inside to outside" state of mind, and vice versa.

Why is it that some individuals can only work while under pressure, and others fall to pieces? How is pressure generated? How is pressure utilized to "control" states of mind, to shift from one state to another? In an earlier chapter (Paul 1981; see Chapter 4), I had quoted the *Oxford English Dictionary*'s definition of pressure, which strongly suggests many elements of the birth experience and reflects the archaic meanings of words close to their origins as having real purchase when describing molding, torture (peine forte et dure), pushing one's way into a space, etc. It is another example of a phenomenon I have described before (Paul and Carson, 1976; see Chapter 2) in which the unconscious meaning of a word is closer to its archaic usage. In the instance of the translation of the word "pressure," I have relied on both my countertransference experience and the patient's use of the term.

To return to the above questions, one simple, yet exceptionally frequent means of elevating mental pressure, is to wait until the last moment, or procrastinate, before engaging in a task. This increases the sense of "pressure" and renders the experience obligatory. The motivation is to get the job done (over with) and the individual experiences an intense pressure often associated with anxiety. The motive force can be the pressure that is generated, which seems to be the primary way that action is initiated. Can this be a vestige of the initiation of action by the uterine pressure on a fetal body as propulsive force? This pressure can be achieved by procrastination, which also has the effect of arousing considerable pain in those around the individual, so that they are provoked to action in an attempt to force the procrastinating individual. Along with procrastination, a variant on this theme, can be either not allowing enough time by having too much to do in too little space to be able to effectively carry out the job. Not starting on time, or delay, is different from packing the time space with too much, but the effect is similar in that it leads to a sense of pressure. It will be immediately recognized that one frequently observes these patterns in every area of a person's life, and that their lives are primarily marked by pressure. A variant of this phenomenon is overextension-undercapitalization, whatever the medium. This often extends to a constant financial pressure and eventual failure, but this combination, although readily recognizable, is exceptionally commonplace. Although the examples given are financial, this description of overextension-undercapitalization is by no means limited to that sphere.

I referred in an earlier example to the process of "getting in deeper" which appears as "greed" superficially. The problem is linked to the intolerance of the mental pain that occurs with the recognition of the effects of the overextension and undercapitalization. Rather than to reduce the extension, there is a compulsion to extend further into a new venture which involves acquisition of something else, removes the attention from the previous problem, which was too painful to remain in contact with, hence, splitting and overextension. Eventually, as the expression states, a person is "spread too thin" and is pushed or motivated to act by the pressure created by the problems which must exist as a result of inattention. Inattention, and failure to maintain proper accounting (record keeping or notation of the facts) come as a result of being intolerant to the pain evoked by the difficulties associated with the problem at hand.

A typical example is as follows: a patient opened a restaurant which, after a while, was doing poorly because, although there was a proper market the management was left to another person who was not closely supervised. When later it was discovered that the restaurant was failing, rather than correct the problem at hand, the patient acquired a larger, much more elaborate restaurant by forming limited partnerships with other investors. The establishment of the second and succeeding projects (getting in deeper) created even greater financial pressure, which was felt physically as a pressure around the head and upper body. In succeeding months, other ventures were added similarly in response to discovering a difficulty in the situation at hand. The patient felt surrounded by interminable pressures and problems which he described as "constant crises," "emergencies," "fires to be put out." No action was taken out of desire, but only when the pressure from a particular sector of the mind became great enough to demand an action. The individual was surrounded by pressures which had to be answered and discharged, or the patient was subject to threat called "crisis," meaning to separate, or "emergency," which is related primarily to the "threat" of emerging.

The hallmark of the experience is the sense of being under and sur rounded by constant pressure, which has every mark of being a strong remnant of memory from the prenatal state where birth is to be avoided at all costs. The person can never stop because the problems "catch up to them." A method of juggling develops which is simply an evasion to hide the undercapitalization. This relationship holds, whether one has a business metaphor, or another form of activity. This is mistakenly called "greed," but can be seen to have its roots in prenatal life organized to avert a crisis or impending disaster.

This series of factors partially creates the phenotype of the experience in which one never has enough and the problem of the sense of frustration is approached by attempting to get more and more of something, that is, a quantitative rather than qualitative approach. The addition of more quantity simply adds more pressure, resulting in expansion-explosion. To say that someone is greedy in this context misses the point of the difficulty, which involves their attempt to operate from a primitive, prenatal state. This can be easily recognized as so-called "manic" style. What I want to emphasize as the invariant is the sense of pressure.

So far, I have concentrated on life-style, or patterned qualities of external behavior, which lead to pressure without describing the use to which the pressure is put, except for motivation and initiation by obligation.

Intrapsychic Induction of Mental Pressure

Pressure can also be induced by self-attack, especially by the choreographed use of cruelty. A typical pattern in a 35-year-old male patient involves initial attacks on the self, "it was not any good anyway"; secondly, a repetition in greater degrees of self-attack quite out of proportion to reality; thirdly, the continued chipping away by the cruel conscience eventuating in gradual discouragement and demoralization. Subsequently, there is erosion of thinking capacity and inability to utilize effective judgment. By then there is unopposed takeover by the cruel conscience and/or psychotic part of the personality with frequent violence or impulsion to hostile action. Continuous breakdown follows.

In this situation all "rejections" stimulating this cycle are perceived as cruelty. Violence can be a function of phantasies of punishment originally linked to the confusion resulting from mental pain being perceived as punishment. Violence can also be a function of experience of the psychotic part of the personality that is deliberately and consciously attacking for the purpose of destructiveness. I include this cycle because it can be observed so frequently in many patients and it leads to explosive rage, which destroys mental functioning. Pressure exceeds the containment threshold and leads to explosion. This destructive cycle is quite typical of the switch from mania to depression and is associated with intense pressure.

I have had a patient who directed an intense force of hatred in a cycle similar to the above description at me for years as a means of effecting a powerful barrier between himself and myself. Typically sessions were missed or seriously compromised by being 30 to 40 minutes late and the kind of cruel diatribe described above would lead to explosive hate and threats of leaving or physical violence if I said anything. I was designated the victim of this cruelty and was supposed to have become depressed which, of course, I did, time and again, before I realized that he was showing me what he experienced when he was alone, and that I represented the nonpsychotic part of his personality. These attacks were mitigated with interpretations of that latter point so that thinking and cooperation would be initiated again to the point of pressure. Bion pointed out that thinking is a process developed to handle the pressure of thoughts (Bion, 1962). When the pressure mounted as a result of the patient's being able to have thoughts, it was the hideous attack that I have previously described that convinced both of us to go no further. The trigger of the attack was the sense of pressure and movement generated by thinking. The attack to produce the barrier between himself and myself, or he and himself, as a cooperative analytical pair, was to put a stop to the thinking process, leading to change, pressure, and the sense of movement associated with birth very similar to the descriptions of Vera by Piontelli (1988). In this instance, pressure could be used to stop thinking by the psychotic rage directed at the thinking part of either the self or other.

Another patient, a 40-year-old surgeon, directed merciless hatred towards his wife and demoralized her continuously in a manner that was quite terrifying. He was hoping that she would leave him, but knew that she would not, which fired his cruelty further. The sessions were severely restricted with excessive formality, and frequent cancellations. However, there was the continuous presence of real development in his life, with many measures of success being attributed to our work, which when recognized as development then led to the cruelty which stopped his functioning. He was obsessed with money and terrified unreasonably about not having it, especially considering his exceptionally high income and sound, conservative management of finances.

Not all effects of pressure are brought on by its augmentation. To demonstrate the effect of diminution of pressure on thinking and feeling, I will report a dream five years into the analysis of this same surgeon. The dream was in three parts:

1. *I am in a chateau, but there is a storm causing the river beneath it to rise. My Uncle Nate was there.*
2. *Suddenly I was in a subway car coming through the chateau resort area.*
3. *It was the Day of Atonement, Yom Kippur, getting ready for Kol Nidre. There was a big congregation of people and a wedding canopy was set up. People were getting married within the congregation during the Yom Kippur service. I say, "You can't get married on Yom Kippur." I knew the brother of the bride, a "jerk" who had a brown velvet suit on. In the congregation, there are groups of eight to ten orchestras, each with their own directors, and at a signal, they all got up and played at the same time, the same song or piece. But each concertmaster was leading his own group. At the chateau, a lady fell down with a seizure. I reluctantly attended her. Maybe that is the false alarm. Then a black baby was abandoned whose father was white. The girl that I saw in consultation last night was Jamaican. I know, he associated, that the dream was stimulated by his wife and family leaving town. "I can breathe, there is room to move and breathe, and the pressure is off. I felt like a weight was lifted off when I dropped them off at the airport."*

When I heard this dream, I was shocked at both its complexity and beauty. There had never been anything remotely like it in the work, only laundry lists of complaints, worries about money, practice and a few dreams, which were terse and highly concrete. The dreams were without associations. In the work, it was revealed that the chateau was the womb, which was represented as breaking the amniotic "bag of waters" and the attendant fears of drowning (Uncle Nate) being a reference to birth, as well as the subway car coming through and out. He is aware of marriage, or linking, occurring between sectors of his mind when he is in the outside state. The Yom Kippur service stood for the at-one-ment, or fusion, along with the awareness of loss or concern demonstrated by the anxiety about the baby's abandonment. Separation, then, first begins with birth and its attendant fears of death. There is a representation of the analyst, "the jerk in the velvet suit" (I wore a velvet sport jacket), and the process was felt to be a harmonious linking up of mental sectors in a coordinated way.

This was the "thinking" and awareness that he was keeping at bay by the maintenance of pressure through worry and attacking hatred to maintain the "divorce" in his marriage, and between he and himself. The "divorce" meant that he would not be born and hence would never suffer abandonment or death. The analysis was also represented by the marriage conducted by the reflection and thought symbolized by the use of the Yom Kippur service.

I report this dream especially to demonstrate a relationship between pressure and the attack on thinking, and depressurizing as a stimulus for the process of thinking. One can see, then, that if there were a means to institute pressure, either internally or externally, one could regulate or control the process of thinking. By increasing the pressure, one could inhibit the thinking process.

To clarify this point a bit more, a similar patient, a 35-year-old single lawyer, dreamt of flashlights and seeing big bears and little bears. This dream related to recognizing his feelings and "bearing them" and the awareness of his mind being illuminated by the analysis. When I interpreted this, he both understood and agreed. Suddenly, his mind filled with a panoply of negative fantasies, all generating pressure. There were Internal Revenue Service attacks, and deployment of Motor Vehicle hassles, which produced pressure, frustration, and a full stop. He said,

> After the "motion" that took me a long time to do (a legal motion) I felt relieved, but to go back to the non-thinking job, part of me feels relieved to do something that requires me no pressure or thinking, but there is a conflict, because I do want to think. You are right, I did play back the "tape" about the IRS and the DMV. It was almost as if I was viewing myself thinking about doing an automatic familiar task requiring no concentration, like an assembly line.

The point was to stop everything, to go on automatic, to stop thinking, then, stop the motion, apply the brakes, establish a motion, so this stopping and starting is typical of the attempt to regulate the sense of pressure and motion which is induced by thinking. The attack is organized to demoralize, or terrorize, to stop motion, and decrease pressure. But now, we can see a further problem associated with the analysis of these individuals addicted to pressured lives. When they begin to slow down and to reduce the pressure enough to begin to move, especially noted by a development of their thinking, feelings emerge which are quite painful and the ensuing development of the phenomenology of the paranoid-schizoid and depressive positions can begin to emerge. This often gives rise to a flood of feelings which can be overwhelming and is stopped by the use of these "braking fantasies." "Braking fantasies" are my way of describing in action terms a fantasy meant to slow or stop a process. These are not symbolic, although they may seem to be, often involving primitive puns, like the one about the "motion." This is often what is meant by coming back into "control" after having been out of control. Psychic movement or development of either thinking or feeling can frequently be associated with the severe anxiety which is defined as going mad, while what is actually occurring is a significant process of development.

Chapter 7
Practical Psychoanalytic Epistemology

In this chapter fundamental distinctions between fact, opinion, and interpretation are considered in the context of their importance to decision making. Special emphasis is given to the exploration of states of mind organized by "induced" affects and phantasies often used in the service of propaganda elaborated in relation to primitive aspects of the personality. The distinction between "induced" phantasy and direct transformation of sense data into experience is of deep practical importance to the establishment of the psychoanalytic process as well as the broader questions as to the nature of "truth" and "falsehood." Clinical examples are presented in the service of clarifying the problems of the patients' recognition of their own approach to the truth. This chapter approaches the problem of the distinction between simulated and "real" experience.

> There's a line between love and fascination, that's hard to see on an evening such as this for they both give the very same sensation when you're under the magic of a kiss.

These lyrics by Ned Washington describe the problem one has in making a distinction between states of mind which produce the same sensation even though their meaning may be quite different. The ballad, "My Foolish Heart," goes on, "for this time it isn't fascination, or a dream that will fade and fall apart, it's love, this time it's love, my foolish heart." This "heartmind" then cannot distinguish between a dream (a self-generated form of evoked experience) and love which is a function of an object relation, i.e., experience coming from another person outside the recipient who is the receiver of the love transmissions. The determination of the distinction between these different states of mind is of considerable practical importance beyond heuristic denotation.

This chapter will deal with the differentiation between the formation of delusion and the fundamental approach to the truth. (Questions about how simulated states of mind are organized versus the experience of uncertainty and vulnerability to direct object related experience are considered in the light of the development of meaning.)

Practical epistemology is presented as an indispensable psychoanalytic tool for the understanding of judgment and the decision making process. In this investigation, the relations between fact, opinion, and interpretation will be considered.

W.R. Bion (personal communication, 1975) said, "A feeling is as close as a fact as you are ever likely to get in psychanalysis." From a scientific point of view, this may seem ambiguous. A feeling can be produced in a way which is induced by the use of a repetitive phantasy. This "fact" is the "same" fact-feeling which is induced by direct contact with the sensuous world. It is obvious that the feeling state coming from an autostimulatory origin and a direct sensuous origin can appear the same to an observer and the person who experiences the feeling directly. How then do we distinguish between an experience which is a simulation of an external experience and one which is directly sensuous (outside in) when the product appears so similar. We live in a world of increasing simulation of experience through computers, artificial intelligence, as well as a dizzying array of induced experiences from pornography to technical video games. We are dealing with nothing less than the fundaments of the accrual of meaning. What kinds of "facts" we are dealing with when we consider direct sensuous versus simulated experience makes a critical difference in the establishment of the accuracy of our interpretations. On the accuracy of interpretation may depend the future of the human species.

Bion, in his characteristic way, drew attention to what now seems an obvious point but which has powerful significance: that the interpretation does not change the facts.

A 42-year-old woman came to analysis for marital problems. She was generally despondent, not only about the difficulty she had with her husband, which resulted in a failure of emotional and sexual relations, but also an increasing sense of isolation and alienation from life in general. She had had a longstanding hostile relationship in which she had been out of contact with her feelings for years and felt she had a poor relationship with her children. She had lived in this state of mind for well over 20 years, and had a series of obsessional and autostimulatory mechanisms which kept her in a state of emotional isolation. She acted out of contact with her feelings, as far as she could tell. She experienced herself as a machine and attempted to live by the standards dictated by a primitive and tyrannical conscience, giving her the illusion of being inorganic, rather like a piece of steel.

The domination of the patient's mind by an imperious, tyrannical and primitive part of the personality, had a long history of organization and was associated with early trauma as a result of severe somatic pathology in the first year of life, which resulted in isolation from maternal contact and produced an elaboration of a set of defenses against contact, the details of which are not important to the development of the story. Nonetheless, the patient, having been dominated by this tyrannical and stereotyped form of cruel conscience, operated in a way to make things occur according to the dictates of her conscience produced in her mind either by an internal visual fantasy, or by a fantasy of some kind of perfection in which she had to live up to the standards or else punish herself. These are all familiar narcissistic defenses which had evolved to a self-stimulatory encapsulated state in which it was impossible for her either to listen or to really talk to another human being, evident in the transference by her deletions and lack of contact palpable in the sessions.

A significant problem which the patient came with had to do with a serious neck problem initiated by an automobile accident, which involved a cervical disc and about which the patient had been in doubt for a considerable amount of time as to what to do about the situation. She had consulted a number of orthopedic surgeons, chiropractors, and neurosurgeons, all yielding a variety of opinions, most of which centered around the inadvisability of doing surgery because of the risk of failure. She hoped simply that she would be able to strengthen herself and that the situation would magically disappear or she would be able to undergo a natural cure by simply leaving the process to change by aging. This had not worked and she suffered increasing cervical instability, such that movements were very difficult for her, causing severe pain. These symptoms disturbed her capacity for work, and she was unable to have social interactions because of her extreme discomfort. Gradually, she used these symptoms as a means of isolating herself from people, including her husband.

In the analytic work there was a gradual development in the direction of establishing emotional contact in which isolating mechanisms became clear. Gradually the analytic work was able to penetrate her defenses which required a direct and confrontative approach. This procedure enabled her to listen to the interpretations and following that, she began to listen to herself. A steady process of analysis of the omnipotent mechanisms over a period of two years enabled the patient to come into emotional contact and realize that she was not going to magically change the situation.

As a result of analysis of these fantasies of omnipotence, she was able to seek consultation and had a series of complicated CT scans (computer tomography) and myelograms of the cervical spine which revealed complicated disc pathology and considerable calcification of the bone outlets from the vertebrae as a result of increasing arthritis in the area. The question then was whether or not the situation could be improved by surgery.

At this point the patient had a conscious decision to make. She did research in the area and conducted a serious inquiry. After having realized that omnipotent mechanisms had failed, she sought the advice of numerous experts who were all reputed to have extensive reputations in this area of specialized spine surgery. The data on the CT scans had been similar. The different versions of the CT scans were in enough agreement so that when they were compared with each other, the radiographic evidence was similar enough so that she was able to discover that the same data (radiographic) produced a completely different set of interpretations by a series of orthopedic surgeons with a consequent divergence of opinion as to what ought to be done about the circumstance. The patient thought that this was not only based on a difference in radiographic evidence, but also a basic difference in skill levels and self-confidence in the surgeons involved. The patient continued her inquiry and gradually an awareness emerged that there were two essential opinions. One opinion was to leave the situation alone, which she had followed in the past by one set of examinations, and another by a prominent orthopedist at a major university hospital who told her quite clearly that surgery was indicated and that he felt that she could be significantly helped and that the downside risk of failure was extremely low.

When the unconscious problems having to do with the magical expectations, obsessional thought and omnipotent mechanisms emerged into consciousness, she brought them under reasonable control. She was then suddenly faced with a decision for which she had previously been incapable of assuming conscious responsibility.

It became evident that a decision is, in fact, a conscious process in which the result and outcome is unknown and that, in fact, as a decision is made, it means by definition that one cannot know the outcome at the time the decision is made. Then the question as to how to make judgments about the myriad sets of information from the variety of different sources, including radiologists and surgeons, were to be assessed and organized in such a way as to be able to allow her to make what she would consider a responsible decision.

On this point, it became clear that there were profound distinctions between matters of interpretation of the same basic evidence. The same set of radiographic facts that have a variety of different interpretations can lead to a variety of different opinions about what action to take. How to sort this out became the primary consideration. What she did realize was that in terms of her experience of her own observations and her state of mind there were certain consistent patterns of facts that she could note. Her neck was continually unstable, and she was in a considerable amount of pain. She could not do a variety of exercises and was considerably immobilized. This reduction of activity had a profound effect on her life both in terms of depressed mood and isolation, and that it was not simply a matter of her using "psychosomatic excuses." These then were facts. Parenthetically, it needs to be developed here that the notion of "psychosomatic" was used in a moral context, as if it was the same as getting away with something or malingering. The "interpretation" of "psychosomatic" came from the cruel conscience disguised as the "internal analyst" who attacks the perception of a physical fact coming from feeling that now is interpreted as some sort of a mental fact in order to be gotten rid of, so that it does not have to be taken into account. In this way the person can evade reality, turn it into a kind of fantasy of a mental process and bring it to a psychoanalyst in order to interpret the entire problem away. There is a kind of delusional security gained by turning something real into something imaginary and then subjecting the process to the services of what Bion (1962) described as minus K.

With the gradual interpretation of these particular phenomena, the situation became more of a conscious bit of analysis, or rather a much neglected area in the field of psychoanalysis, that is the analysis of the *conscious.* That is, how to make distinctions between matters of opinion, and matters of fact. This is what Bion was referring to when he articulated the notion of practical epistemology and its importance in not only making philosophical distinctions between categories and classes of experience on the basis of pure intellectual pursuit, but rather that psychoanalysis in this sense has as its goal a primary orientation which must lead to action or the analysis is of no practical use.

The consistent observation of feeling her own physical instability and pain served as a compass point which the interpretations on clear recognition did not change. The radiographic interpretations, her visits to the surgeons, or her visits to me as an analyst, did not change the physical symptomatology. It then became clear that interpretation *per se* does not change facts as is a general point. It is of great significance that there can be the illusion that if one makes an accurate interpretation, the act of interpreting then removes the problem. She was able to discover the fact that that was not the case and by accepting the realization that interpretations do not change facts, she was then able to accept the problem of having to act on information about which she was uncertain in an area in which there were opposing opinions about the same set of radiographic evidence. This evidence served as the substrate of information for having to make a decision as to what she would do: whether she would actually take the advice of the surgeon who emphasized the downside risk being low and the likelihood of a surgery being successful, versus those who were advising waiting.

The patient experienced a great deal of relief in the session as she was able to recognize what the issues were and what the actual decision was then based on. She was then able to make a decision to go ahead with the surgery, even though she could not know the outcome. She was considerably anxious about it but felt a definite depressive concern. She was sad and felt grateful toward me in the session and was able to feel a real sense of softness and gentleness. There was a sense of hope with the acknowledgment that there were agents of real help aside from omnipotent phantasies on which she could rely. I could perceive a vast affective change in the patient, instead of being rigid and speaking in a stereotyped, mechanical way, there was suddenly a highly sensitive person with great sophistication who had realized that she did have the courage to make a decision based on the realization of that which she had to consider.

A 52-year-old professional man came to analysis for a variety of complaints, including marital difficulties, incipient divorce and poor relations with his children. He complained bitterly about having a violent temper, becoming enraged to the point of not being able to understand what was being said to him, and felt that he did not care who was with him. He simply isolated himself and could not tolerate the presence of other people. He treated his children, wife, and himself rather in the same way.

He spoke in a kind of cross sounding, raspy, harsh voice that was scattered and he seemed to pay very little attention to what he said. He paid very little attention to what I said as well. As a result there was not very much meaningful interaction possible in the session, leading to a very peculiar situation in which one had the feeling in the countertransference of quasi frustration and indifference beginning to develop. A feeling of a deeply despairing pain coming as a result of not being listened to or regarded was evident. Thus, a situation occurred in which I and the patient were talking, he was not listening, and I was becoming convinced that it was rather a bad idea to listen. I drew his attention to this state of affairs. He said that he "discounts" the meaning of verbal communication, and assumes that people simply do not mean what they say and that there is no point to paying attention. He put forward the idea that he could never understand where my interpretations came from. He had assumed that they came out of the air or my "imagination" and that probably interpretations did not make any difference anyway since in fact he was not particularly concerned himself, that whatever occurred would occur by magical means if it were to happen at all. The idea that he might be able to understand where the interpretations came from if he were aware of what he said himself was an idea that had never occurred to him. It seemed to him that it was extraordinarily hostile of me to suggest paying attention and that there was a requirement for him to listen not only to himself but to myself as well. In this particular transferential situation the patient could not tell the difference between an opinion, an interpretation or a fact. Drawing attention to facts in the session made no difference at all, in the sense that he could not distinguish an event which had actually happened, and which was true, from one which had not.

In this instance I am using as a definition of opinion, according to the shorter *Oxford English Dictionary*, "a judgment resting on grounds insufficient for complete demonstration; belief of something as probable or as seeming to our own mind to be true. What is generally thought about something." The *Oxford English Dictionary* defines *interpretation* as follows: 1) to expand the meaning of; to render clear or explicit, to elucidate, to explain. 2) formerly, to translate; b) to explain to oneself; c) inferential, constructive.

These differential points are quite important to define, in that the practical process of making a decision or understanding the meaning of an experience depends very much on whether one thinks that something is a matter of opinion, interpretation, or fact. These distinctions would have greater meaning, if one expected to have one's own mental processes lead to something. The notion that one could think about something, process information in one's mind by a sophisticated method of judgment or by considering a matter over a period of time in which delay was possible, produced discomfort in the patient. Regarding contingent possibilities, weighing opinions, or considering matters of interpretation of the same set of facts from different perspectives was a foreign experience. He simply operated by reaction, a kind of instantaneous reactivity which substituted for thinking. Therefore, the notion of utilizing the processes of mature judgment and then subsequently putting that resultant judgment into action was something impossible for him. Moreover, severe impoverishment of interpersonal contact was manifested by his inability to listen to himself or to other people. His capacity for attention was severely restricted and therefore his capacity to make distinctions such as I mentioned above between fact. opinion, and interpretation was impossible. Thus, learning from experience was severely impaired.

Another patient, a 48-year-old male attorney, displayed a particular element of his personality that opposed and perceived the analyst consistently as the enemy in defiance of all the facts. The patient was in his sixth year of analysis and had developed a markedly improved relationship with his children which had previously been dysfunctional, and had acknowledged considerable benefit from the analytic work. He had been unable to "feel," and now he experienced deep feelings and was able to tolerate the separation from his wife with whom he had had a primary infantile relation. After considerable work and experimentation he formed a close relationship with a woman. His previous inability to tolerate delay or frustration which were causes for his business failure as a result of his incapacity for attention had developed sufficiently so that he considered the analysis to have helped him significantly in that his thinking processes were considerably clearer.

There is a bit of him that opposes and perceives the analyst consistently as an enemy in defiance of the facts. He will say *anything.* Even if it is demonstrated as a lie, it is unimportant to him. He will *exaggerate* the lie and repeat it over and over again in a kind of violent way. He becomes shocked at the awareness of this distortion when it is pointed out to him that it doesn't seem to matter whether the facts are paid attention to. This bit of him seems to say whatever it likes, no matter what the conditions, and leads to the establishment of a mental set, coordinated to produce a particular state of mind. The state of mind involves a kind of nonlocation in space, as if to say I am not at place X, rather than I am at this point. Thinking is utilized in this particular instance in the services of what Bion (1962) has referred to as minus K. This nonlocation leads to a particular organization of feeling. A is a nonlocation in space, and B is a particular feeling that is associated with that. This "thought-feeling organization" is repeated *ad infinitum.* The communication to the patient through a propagandistic part of himself is that nothing has changed because he is behaving the same, and there is produced in others the same attitudes in relation to his "personality." In this instance the patient's lodestone is the "know-it-all," opinionated, loud, clumsy, enclosed state of mind that says anything, does not listen, interrupts, talks on and on, rails and complains about everything that is not the way the patient would like to be. He puts forward a form of primary negativity which leads to frustration, anger, rage and depression, and then repeats, and repeats, *ad infinitum,* without the circumstances being true. This produces a kind of orientation of familiarity that can be plotted on the negative side of a set of mental coordinates. The peculiar situation is that in this instance one is struck by the repetition which leads to a state of affairs that produces a feeling state which is highly recognizable and consistent so that it serves as a primary organizer in the mind of the individual, and acts perversely as a kind of comfort. The feeling organization that this particular organization of phantasy produces is real.

It is a "fact" such that the perceptible sensation which is produced in the mind is replicable over and over again. This leads to a considerable epistemologic problem to define the distinction between a particular organization of feeling that is produced from inside by means of this auto-stimulatory organization stemming from a primitive part of the personality versus that of an object related, open state of mind in which experience comes from the outside and has a direct effect on the mind of the individual. The primary difference with which one must be concerned would be the difference between a simulation of experience and the feeling of an object related, actual experience in the external world outside as having occurred. This differentiation is extremely important in order to sort out distortions of reality resulting from transmissions from the psychotic part of the personality and/or primitive archaic conscience, acting as a source of propaganda. Visual fantasies, feelings, organized dreams, sound and tone can be utilized rather like the artistic function of a film director organizing a state of affairs in which the individual is "convinced" of the "meaning" of his experience, especially as a result of being repetitive and consistently able to be reproduced. Therefore, the differentiation between that state of affairs and the organization of feeling coming from the outside is a psychoanalytic problem of very great proportions.

I had the experience in my own analysis of considerable confusion when in the presence of a defined feeling evident in the session. Bion would refer to "a feeling being as close to a fact as you are ever likely to get in psychoanalysis." This particular analytic statement opened up a world of questions which I am still having difficulty formulating but are nevertheless clearly present in a form which continues to be revealed. What is the difference between a feeling and a simulated feeling? What language do we use to describe the difference?

The *Oxford English Dictionary* defines *fact* as: 1) a thing done or performed, (a) an action, deed; 2) something that has really occurred or is the case; hence, a datum of experience as distinguished from conclusions.

A painter in his forties had the following dream:

A woman was teaching a class at the university. She was highly respected and adopted a confident demeanor of both humor and authority. One had the feeling that she was not to be crossed without the veneer of humor bring splintered for her truthful underlayer, a menacing dictatorial quality, evidenced by the formed blast of her voice, filling its column full throated but having burnished edges. A collimated armor-piercing packet of energy resulted, emerging in jactated lurches and ricocheting off the surfaces of the room, producing dangerous and ominous tones. She was elaborating a theory having to do with language, perhaps linguistics. Perhaps fifty young men and women populated the lecture hall. They sat at children's desks and were writing respectfully as she spoke. When she had finished, she announced that payment of additional fees were required, and I felt a sudden pain. A combination of rage, fear and tears were rounded up as though they were unruly children in the hands of a disciplined adult. I was frightened, but the children wanted to attack, to scream, to rage, to retaliate, but I spoke knowing it was as if I was defending against my likely risk of suffering harm. I held them quietly and said, "You are asking the class to pay you in addition to the tuition?" She said yes and, although taken aback, she pushed forward like an animal in a headwind. She was "discovered" and angry. She knew her reputation was in danger but said, with easy authority, that the extra payment was the custom, and that was that. She collected her notes and, as she left the room, told me in front of the group that I could decide if I was to continue. It was clear that we hated each other, she for being crossed, questioned and exposed, and I for her lying perversion. She was cruel, no doubt of it. The others nervously and hurriedly gathered their belongings and left, but with a sense of terror, I ran after a freckle-faced redhead of about nineteen. Sharon was an English major and was serious. I said to her, "Look, was I rude?" She replied, "Yes, or so it could have certainly appeared. I don't think that was the best of your ideas and certainly was poor judgment." I said, "But it was a lie, unfair, misrepresenting the truth." Sharon looked at me with a sidelong sense of dismissal and said, "You'll never know the difference and neither will anyone else." I knew I had not studied for the exam, but nonetheless I disagreed and defied her. Fears permeated my being and I spoke, guarding against the emergence of the feeling, as though an animal would respond by snapping at the prey. I was left to nurse the depression and terrific sadness. I had no good feeling left. I had survived, but I could never go back nor achieve her "help" in creating images, sounds or other sensory distractions. I now had an enemy. The lines were drawn. But it was clear I was crushed I had no choice, and the unpleasant feeling of no interest in the truth. Since obviously I knew

> *what it was and that it was unobtainable; Sharon, goddess of reason, had told me so. I knew she was deluded, but what was the use of talking? At that time, I had not the ability to confront her, and I was left alone without companions. Neither the liars, who were my former protectors, nor the intellectuals, who were egoistic dictators, and not my Sharon, who had incredibly sexy legs, only flawed by heavy freckling. She was an Irish Rhode Island Red who disappeared down the hall. I knew I was in trouble. I would like to approach the truth, but I don't like the idea I'm going to die, not even a little. I'm no longer rewarded by the image of blacksweatered intellectuals smoking Gauloises and being one or another edition of the "existential hero." The deep, grieving sadness could not be quelled. There is no way out, no exit.*

An extremely well mannered and articulate young lawyer appeared calm, but was furious. He had had a dream in which a turtle, not a tortoise, was present. The turtle was the "cheap variety," one bought and found in plastic boxes with artificial moss in five and dime stores. He knew it was fragile and had to be protected, so he placed it in his shirt pocket. His associations involved the turtle being slow, but he was "not" listening to the "hype" of this voice and voices that he constantly hears that are attacking anything beautiful. These voices produce a sense of intense pain. In fact, he said, he had heard Pavarotti the night previously, which sent chills up and down his spine. Then he was suddenly frightened when he associated that I would think he was a name dropper. He noted the immediate criticism by an attacking part of himself and then said, "I don't know anything about opera." Then there was an attack again as he slowed down. He said he did not know the future. "I used to think I did." Suddenly, at that point, there seemed like a huge dose of "drugging numbness" that I was able to recognize in the countertransference and I had everything I could do to maintain my state of alertness. The drugging interfered with the impact of my interpretation about the intensity of feelings of beauty causing very intense pain and, at that point, he said, "I feel the need to do nothing for awhile. I don't know how long it has been since I looked at clouds and sky. I'd get bored if I did," he said. I interpreted that the boredom was the effect of this "drug" that he was able to use to knock out his feelings. He said,

> Yes, it works in two steps. It says, "You can't just lie here. You have things to do. You have to pay the bills. You have to return phone calls, wash the car." Why can't I just lie here? "No, no, no. Can't waste time." It's like

> then I hear a lyric "take a kayak to Quinsy or Nyack, let's get away from it all." So it is the sort of thing that (1) you hear, "here's a life, follow the orders, pay the bills, and do what you're told." That's what I did for many years. But then there's another life that comes as a result of the feeling and the anesthesia of it. It's, (2) "I'm bored. No interest in anything." Then the defense against that is (3) "Let's take a kayak to Nyack," which are radically different ways of living that are derived essentially from the same experience.

I interpreted that in rhythm A (1) his experience related to a manic march in which there was "no time to say hello, goodbye, I'm late, I'm late, I'm late" that is, a very, rapid, clipped, speedy moving on. Rhythm B (2) felt to him as though time had been massively slowed down to a dragging quality, almost yielding the quality of a recording played at half speed which then resulted in this drugging anesthesia. Then the C rhythm (3) is an escape from that, which is the "Let's take a kayak to Nyack" seduction. First, there is the manic march and then the drag that comes as a result of that, which then prompts this C view, that is the "kayak to Nyack" view. "Don't be ridiculous, we can't get away from it all, that's a half baked fantasy." The same experience can yield three different speeds or rhythms of speech. When I say the same experience, I mean that defenses against a particular experience of feeling is evidenced in three different velocities of speech which allow for different feelings to emerge.

In this example, we are making distinctions between derivatives of the same fantasy, which lead to different affects dominating at different times with different results. For example, it makes a considerable difference as to whether one interprets one's own experience as being bored when one, in fact, is drugged. One never knows what the "drug" is "drugging," yet it's clear here that the drug is drugging the sense of beauty that he experienced having listened to Pavarotti which produced chills up and down his spine and made him feel very deeply. That was extremely uncomfortable and provoked massive criticism.

The criticism then was so painful that, in order to block out the feeling associated with the sense of deep beauty, he drugged himself or anesthetized himself to avoid the pain of the criticism. That was the secondary response. The tertiary response, Rhythm C, was associated with the song fantasy, "Let's take a kayak to Nyack, let's get away from it all," a standard song which seemed to move him out of the psychic space associated with the painful fantasy.

One of the most painful experiences in psychoanalysis can be the discovery that that which is a recognition of the truth or the approach to the truth is very different from what was previously imagined or anticipated. One is not here simply dealing with the disappointment, which is a natural resultant upon the discovery of false expectation. Although frequently producing rage and consequent depression, if the splitting mechanisms no longer "work," there is also a deepening awareness of a chronic state of mental pain, sadness, loss, and grief that one has to come to this pass without any reassurance of emerging. There is a clear awareness of one's previous false assumptions being not only deluded but ludicrous. There is the further problem that this cause for ridicule is beyond the realm of logical propositions and that a domain of experience has been opened out that has a logic, all right, but it is not Aristotelian. These *painful feelings* do not cease readily. "Interpretations" which had had the effect of the lysis of pain no longer do the same work. Again here, it is important to note that the *interpretations* do not change the facts (of these painful experiences). While *understanding* indubitably makes possible use of greater logical skills, there is diminished infusion of omnipotent streams of thought to "alter" feeling (upregulate painful affect). The resulting logical analysis is usually discovered to have greater accuracy. This does not produce relief because it has become obvious that that on which one has depended upon for support (lies, exaggerations, upregulating fantasies) are damaging to accuracy but at least produce relief. It would seem that one would be faced with a choice between accuracy (a derivative of truth) and relief of pain.

Patients are rarely pleased or grateful with this state of affairs. The question of enmity occurs with increasing frequency. Is the truth our friend? Does the truth really set one free? Does the analyst, who has obviously produced this change, have friendly intentions? Does he know what he is doing? It is a frequent observation that many patients do not have a prejudice in favor of the truth. When we analyze someone who deeply favors lies, I think one can practically consider this a sign of profound fear of change brought about by the truth. If this person is pushed to continue, they often become hostile because they feel they are in danger of being brought to death. The linearity of time and the experience of this set of experiences, in addition to the awareness that one's mental tools had never developed properly to investigate accurately, is an unhappy combination. There is no relief in attacking reality because one realizes the foolishness of it, based on *obviously false assumptions,* in addition to the clear realization of the damage done to one's objects as a result. Concern leads, therefore, to a continuous exposure of what has not been resolved, which emerges in painful presence no longer to be split off. The trouble is that one's analyst has brought one there, and this analysis often has led to intense pain. To bring to the analyst further material seems to promise deeper pain, yet to "escape" is worthy of the realization that this escape is only possible by delusion. Ridicule, which is no stranger to the patient, is an extremely frequent accompaniment. Further analysis can bring into focus the destructive effects of this ridicule which may ameliorate the hostile reproach producing clinical depression but leaves the extremely intense pain previously described which has no immediate cure. Here, the inspired beliefs of the past and the vast array of mental drugs available through honed fantasy via advertising, etc., have no immediate effect on the pain any longer. There can be an awareness of the trial of various fantasies to effect change and state of mind. When I refer to honed fantasies, I mean ones which have been "selected" for their efficacy. These honed fantasies are powerful euphoriants, distractors, seducers, sexual exciters, etc. These have been relied upon for the patient's lifetime. Now they are without the use of them.

In considering the means by which fantasy is honed, one must consider the intelligent observing function of an aspect of the mind known variously as the archaic superego and/or primitive superego. I think that the primitive superego is contiguous with Bion's concept of the psychotic-part-of-the-personality. I have observed that one major function of this aspect of the personality is to detect psychic movement. If movement is felt to occur in the "forward direction" toward development, maturation, progress, there are brought into play "defenses" against this imagined danger. These broad categories of psychic change trigger a variety of "honed" fantasies used to dissuade, distract, seduce or, in general, move off the point of engagement that leads to the progress or to awareness of the progress. This "intelligent" awareness (psychotic part or archaic part) "defends" the individual against development, especially those functions which disturb the time arresting fantasies. When linear time is introduced, there is a "recognition of danger" and thereby the initiation of inhibitory fantasies usually involving terror and/or seduction. When more complete inhibition is "required" to stop growth or the perception of change, then drugging occurs, which I have previously elaborated (Paul, 1981; see Chapter 4). This sleepy, drugged anesthesia is very difficult to battle as the *Aeneid* relates (in the death of Palinurus). Psychoanalysis leads to the capacity to conduct a conscious battle against the movement off point by developing the mental strength to conduct vigilant self analysis (required in order to) recognize the interfering fantasies. It becomes clear in the actual sessions that this work of self analysis is required and leads to the question of how much self reliance is required to work through the deflections from contact on one's own.

One can readily see that the job required of the patient is a matter of his capacity or level of development to counteract or contain inhibitory fantasies in order to move forward. This point provides an assay for both "growth" and mental development and also the degree of progress in analysis, and also can serve as a major factor in the consideration of the termination of the analysis, and further, what is meant by analytic success. If we as analysts take the position of favoring maturation and development, we radically oppose the time arresting archaic superego's functions and engage a battle for supremacy.

The notions of "superego" have been brilliantly described by Bion (1962). His point is that this "superior object" asserts its superiority by finding fault with everything.

> The most important characteristic is its hatred of any new development in the personality, as if the new development were a rival to be destroyed. The emergence, therefore, of any tendency to search for the truth, to establish contact with reality and, in short, be scientific, in no matter how rudimentary a fashion, is met by destructive attacks on the tendency and the reassertion of the "moral" superiority (pp. 97-99).

This implies an assertion of what, in sophisticated terms, would be called a moral law and a moral system as superior to scientific law and scientific system. Bion goes on to relate the disintegrating, destructive effect to a phenomenologic description of envy which removes the description from the exclusivity of the moral vertex.

I had mentioned powerful phantasies which act as euphoriants, distractors, seducers, powerful sexual exciters, etc. These have been relied upon for the patient's lifetime. Now, they are without them. There is a special reduction of the effects of a powerful narcotic diminisher of painful sensation and affect and, indeed, all affect. This diminished drugging leads to greater sensation and emotion, but since the anesthesia cannot be turned on as before, now there is consistent presentation to the facts. These patients have frequently built their lives, chosen their friends, related to their objects in a manner banding against the truth. If this was the predominant means by which there could be relations, now there is a sense of fear, disappointment, and extraordinary loneliness. To maintain the previous mode of false relations to outside, allows little pleasure because of the awareness of the process. There can be a true hatred of the process which has brought one to this realization. Frequent attempts to change external relations meet with utter frustration because the analysand is alone with the awareness of the delusion in him/herself and in their fellows. If this is not welcome information to oneself, it would be extremely unlikely that one's friends would find it pleasurable or interesting.

Sadomasochism is a frequent accompanying process in descriptions of addictions to near death (Betty Joseph, 1982), or addictions to misery. Therefore, making the distinction between the pain associated to the addiction to misery and the pain related to the discoveries related to accuracy is very difficult indeed. The addiction to misery can be identified when the fantasies have been recognized which produce the breaking off of contact. If the fantasies employed by the "influencing machine" (Tausk, 1919) archaic superego will involve self-deprecation, self-attack, terror and sadomasochistic "moral" means, then misery is the result, and the addiction to misery serves to stave off the awareness of change in the developmental forward direction. One could just as effectively employ seductive fantasies of a much more pleasurable quality to achieve a similar result. I include the following example to demonstrate the "stopping" or inhibiting function.

A 53-year-old professional woman had the following dream.

> *She was in a college or educational setting and was about to go on a trip to a reunion. A requirement was that a thesis be completed in order to be handed to the ticket agent, who upon receipt of the thesis, would issue the ticket. Many individuals were leaving but, to her shock, the thesis was suddenly gone and the patient had a strong suspicion that this teacher had stolen it to prevent her going to the reunion. She mustered other classmates who had seen her with the thesis, and she summoned the Dean who had the teacher's briefcase searched and her drawers rifled, but no thesis could be found. The Dean therefore considered the corresponding stories of her schoolmates to be hearsay and could not effectively evaluate the evidence. The student was extremely frustrated both at having to try to redo the thesis and at the teacher's cleverness at having stolen the thesis and hidden the evidence so well.*

In the dream, movement is represented by going on a trip to a reunion (development in relation to reuniting; reuniting with split off aspects of the self as well as contact with time). In her associations, a reunion was a unique situation allowing for the comparison of the time periods, the past with the present. One sees how far one has come to the present situation as time is acknowledged and one is forced to "catch up." There is a clear association of the "teacher" with both the one who assigns the task and the thief who wishes to stop the patient's going ahead by theft. This realization was attended by intense anxiety and a desire to leave the consulting room (claustrophobia), to get out into the air. This concern and judgment between the honest assignment of tasks and standards (mature superego function) and the clever theft to prevent progress, both engage sophisticated systems of thought organized into judgment. The "moral" component is clearly noted here, but its accuracy is in doubt. Was the thesis stolen or not?

There are profound feelings of frustration and resentment at the perceived unfairness of the teacher which can be dominating, as they are in the situation described, leading to the profound anxiety and rapid action. The motivation to continue the progress to development is clear as the patient is clearly mustering what is required for reassemblage of the thesis.

Forward and backward movement is linked with progress and inhibition and is observable in the transference by the perception of contact which varies during the session from closeness to avoidance, a rudimentary set of crude coordinates which can be used to establish direction (Paul, 1993; see Chapter 6).

I do not wish to engage the obvious reference to rules of evidence and other procedures of law, but it seems clear that issues of judgment here are likely to have considerable significance if issues of intent are matters of concern and clearly of opinion and interpretation.

The teacher said the witnesses were not "close enough" to the student to see exactly what the writing was on the paper. They could only say that it was the proper size and shape as a thesis. The Dean ruled that this eye witness account was insufficient evidence to rule in favor of the student.

The psychotic part of the personality, or archaic superego, can muster a reasoned approach to oppose change. Crafty, clever, facile tricks are employed which fit within the system of acceptable standards and are used to stop recognition of the facts. The overlap of evidence in relation to its use by both aspects of the personality gives rise to reasonable doubt. This can lead to the stopping of the investigation. The resemblance of the process of analytic "scientific" investigation can be felt to be indistinguishable from criminal investigation (Paul, 1989; see Chapter 5).

Chapter 8

Intonational Elements as Communication in Psychoanalysis

Intonational elements of communication have frequently been overlooked in psychoanalysis, although recently sound qualities are beginning to be investigated in human speech interactions because of powerful discoveries in modern infant research. William Condon, for example, clearly demonstrated that articulate speech has a direct effect in integrating the pattern of gross muscular movement in the one day-old infant, and that the syntactic patterns of speech introduced to the infant have later shaping effects not only on his or her coordinated movements but on the pattern of vocal response organization linked to primitive object relations. Vocal communication is a necessary condition to fulfill this interactive relation, although the response is not dependent on specific language form. Mechanical sounds such as clicks do not produce the coordinated response which is specific to human vocal communication from the first day of life (Condon and Sander, 1974).

Brazelton's recent studies have investigated the complex stereotype of cueing interactive process between mother and infant so that it is quite clear that the connection between the two is established beyond the range of simple anatomy by a complex series of links including visual and auditory elements such as smiling, direct eye engagement and tonal qualities which involve loudness, pitch and sonority (Brazelton, Koslowski, and Main, 1973; Brazelton, 1975).

When one considers the vast complex of factors involved in establishing meanings in human vocal interaction, it is immediately clear that a great deal is dependent on tonal elements in addition to what is actually communicated by words alone. There are considerable difficulties in communicating such qualities, partly because of the inadequacy of verbal language to make fine distinctions that refer to tone. This becomes immediately evident when one reads music and can see that the system of notation is much more highly developed for this purpose. Not only is pitch accurately referred to, based on a standard of physical measurement (A = 440 cycles/second), but dynamics, rate of dynamic shift, intensity, meter, connectedness (legato-staccato), and balance, to name only a few, can be represented and repeated with such a degree of accuracy that we can simulate a Gregorian chant or the atmospheric mood in an eighteenth-century drawing room.

The degree of specificity possible in coloring mood elements is considerable, without altering pitch or dynamics, but by subtle changes in interval voicing so that the same notes in a chord, played simultaneously, will produce an easily recognizable change and receptive response merely by altering one voice in a group of ten while the others are held constant. I mention this to underscore the sensitivity of the auditory discriminative response so that one can define the orchestral effects of Beethoven and Stravinsky instantaneously or recognize the innovations in mood or affective response of voicing patterns organized by an artist such as the late Bill Evans, who has had profound effects on the development of modern keyboard improvisation.

Ezra Pound (1968) was adamant about the inclusion of tonal considerations in one's study of meaning and advocated the study of early Italian song forms and the early works of the troubadours in Languedoc. He insisted that his students should learn to sing the forms because the meaning was established by tonal and rhythmic elements. In his essay, "How to read," he noted that the communication of meaning in poetry was established by three routes. In *phanopoeia*, the casting of images on the mind through language, the route is directed to the mind's eye. *Logopoeia*, the dance of the intellect among the senses, is dependent on the stimulation of a variety of internal mental sense receptors. *Melopoeia*, however, establishes meaning primarily through the sound of the communication, so that theoretically one could understand elements of meaning without understanding the verbal element of the language.

The use of tonal elements to produce a mind set has an ancient heritage. The sounds of shepherds' pipes is indeed different from the piper's call to battle. The march form produces mental effects very different from that stimulated by Strauss.

"Tone of voice" has effects on mind set which are clearly independent of content. In tonal languages such as Chinese or Thai, the same word has five different tonal renditions which produce five different meanings independent of inflection. Some individuals pick out tonal elements almost exclusively to determine meaning, so that one can be surprised that the complex formulation one wished to communicate was experienced as a lullaby or, for that matter, an attack.

I have become more aware of the complexities of sound elements which enter into the establishment of a state of mind. Richard Grove, a professor of music, introduced me to the experience that one could play a melody changing only the voice distribution and produce specific effects on state of mind with great accuracy. I do not think it was only that the tune was "Fly me to the moon." This phenomenon, however, is nothing new to the musician, who can observe these known effects in his audience with pleasure and know how to organize a solo improvisation that will move them through a sequences state of mental changes, which jazz musicians humorously call "cheap tricks." These "tricks" have very benign effects which become desirable to understand as a performer but have an importance considerably beyond this when one remembers that certain mental sets may not be so benign. Listening to Hitler's speeches can be very illuminating in this regard, as an extreme example. Again, this is not a new observation in itself, but it may be wise to consider it when establishing conditions for the communication system in a psychoanalytic setting. How does the patient "play the analyst" and vice versa?

When playing ensemble music or singing part harmony, a balance is required for musical communication. A highly developed form of intense concentration is necessary to attend to one's own part as well as listening to its relation in blending with the group. Timbre, inflection, loudness, and pressure or intensity of voice are varied to "match" the qualities in which there is mutual participation, to ensure an effective blend and a lack of dominance. However, it is frequently desirable to bring out a melody line or to accentuate certain inner voicings (distribution of notes) to change the meaning of a musical communication. These are far too complex to enter into here in detail, but may be profitably considered as a model for vocal balance in an analytic setting. One would not only consider what one wanted to say, then, but also how it was said. In listening, too, one would be advised to pay attention to the quality of sound presented as an additional important source of information in formulating and interpretation.

This kind of listening, then, would involve a powerfully focused beam of attention which would be distributed between listening to one's self and to the other simultaneously. As a result, there is a monitoring of sound quality on a continuous basis on the part of the analyst (Freud, 1912). I think this is somewhat different from the evenly suspended attention which Freud advises, and I find it can profitably be applied to the analytic situation, shifting from one form of attention to the other in order to pick up information from multiple vertices on a simultaneous basis. I do not mean here to deny the importance of the evenly suspended attention of Freud; only to add the form of musical listening which is held in common by ensemble players and is intensely focused.

Utilizing this model as a tool, then, has the profound advantage that one can observe phenomena which can induce variations in the capacity for attention in both members of the analytic pair.

1. Linguistic Considerations

In defining elements of human language, linguists distinguish between verbal, prosodic and paralinguistic features. Taking prosody first: according to the *Oxford English Dictionary*, *prosody* refers to that part of the study of language which deals with the forms of metrical composition; formerly reckoned as a part of grammar and also including phonology or phonetics.

Lyons (1972) mentions intonation and stress as instances of the prosodic features of utterance:

> Every normal English utterance is produced with a particular intonation "pattern" or "contour" which is determined partly by the grammatical structure of the utterance and partly by the attitude of the speaker (as dubious, ironical, surprised, etc.). If two utterances of the same sequence of words differ with respect to their intonation, they would probably be described by linguists as two "different" utterances, rather than as two instances of the same utterance. In English, each word would be pronounced with a certain degree of stress or "emphasis" according to its grammatical function and a variety of other functions including the contextual presuppositions of the utterance, the attitude of the speaker, and so on. If two utterances of the same sequence of words differ in stress, they would probably be described as two different utterances . . . intonation and stress as examples of prosodic features are almost universally regarded as being part of language . . . They are nonverbal: They do not identify or form part of the words of which the utterance is composed and yet they are an essential part of what is commonly referred to as "verbal signals" (pp. 52-53).

Paralinguistic features are described as combinations of physiologically grounded parameters, with pitch, loudness, duration and silence variable in relation to their identification. This restricts the term to features of vocal signals.

Michael Argyle (1972), referring to the description of nonverbal aspects of speech, describes prosodic and paralinguistic features as follows:

> [prosodic signals include] pitch pattern, stress pattern and juncture (pauses and timing) which affect the meaning of sentences and are regarded as true parts of the verbal utterances. Paralinguistic signals include emotions expressed by tone of voice, group membership expressed by accent, personality characteristics expressed by voice quality, speech errors, etc. These nonverbal signals are not closely linked with language, do not have a complex structure and are similar to other expressions of attitudes and emotions (p. 251).

I think that while these nonverbal signals may not be closely linked with language structure, they do have a complex psychological structure, and here psychoanalysts may have something to contribute to the understanding of both prosodic and paralinguistic features of language.

2. Elements in Human Speech Functioning as Forms of Action

In this chapter, I wish to sketch the beginning forms of certain vocal elements in human speech which function primarily as forms of action. The elements of speech themselves, often articulate and symbolic, are used not merely as elements of communication but also with the effect of actions, which I have likened to drug activity because of the experiential qualities described. They are often also used to deflect or stop the communication process. Rhythm will certainly be obvious in the manic patient: rapid bursts of pressured speech coding for avoidance of sadness, awareness of loss or vulnerability. Certain effects such as sadness and love cannot be experienced when the rhythm is too rapid— rather like playing a musical recording at too great a speed. The musical notes in relation to one another are recognizable, but the experience of feeling originally represented is no longer available. If there is to be a communication of joy, however, it cannot be experienced at too slow a velocity. Meltzer (1984) suggests

> [a] two-tiered structure of language, one operating from the depths of the unconscious for the purpose of transmitting states of mind by the operation of projective identification, while the other, more conscious, superimposes words on this deep music for the purpose of communicating information about the outside world (p. 96).

> The great cleavage in the linguistic field is over the issue of whether the primary unit of language is the phoneme (the unit of sound) or the morpheme (the unit of meaning). Those who oppose the phoneme as an artificial unit created by phonologists, on whatever ground they have their argument—psychological, methodological, or theoretical—seem none the less to assume that a unit must he found. The reason for this is apparent, for all linguists seem to assume that language has the primary function of communicating information . . . It is apparent that this is not a model, simile or metaphor, but a statement. It [language] places speaker and listener in relation to one another as tuned instruments (pp. 97-98).

If there is a reaction between speaker and listener requiring attunement, then what if these reactions were within the same individual between parts of the personality, so that the sound quality is communicated internally as well as interpersonally? It is this nonlinguistic, nonsyntactical, nonverbal musical element I wish to extract from the ground qualities of language with specific reference to intonation. What is obviously needed is a system of notation which could be used in lateral communication between analysts in formulating more precise references to these musical elements. In Meltzer's (1984) theory of grammar, there is also a two-tiered system:

> Depth (unconscious) grammar includes the phonemic-morphemic elements of vocalization in all its musical aspects . . . as well as the logical operations of syntax which are implied in the juxtapositions contained in the unconscious phantasy sequence. Surface grammar contains all those modifications of vocalization which the communication of information about the external world requires in order to minimize the many possible forms of ambiguity—and therefore confusion (p. 112).

I am in agreement with Meltzer's notion of an unconscious grammar in reference to his musical elements. I suspect that there are operational musical patterns that have the effect of opening and closing the mind. By closing the mind, I refer to not being able to listen and thereby learn from experience. Some of the musical elements closing the mind include repetitive percussiveness (pounding), monotonous pitch control involving lack of variation, intense pressure of speech and threatening harsh sound. Lullaby-like sounds can also seduce the closure of the mind.

A professional man in his late forties came for psychoanalysis as a result of marital difficulties. He could not understand why he could not tolerate feelings. He had a history of separation from his mother in his first year of life, in which she was reputed to have had a "nervous breakdown." The patient was very frightened and resistant to analysis but came because he "should," although he readily stated that coming was repugnant.

It was soon clear that when he spoke he paid little attention to what he said and although he seemed to listen to interpretations, he noticed that whole sections of my sentences were deleted from his hearing. He would mask this by asking me to repeat interpretations and responded with considerable concern when, upon my showing him the "deletion" from hearing or auditory perception, he could note that he had trouble remembering what he had said as well. Considerable sections of both our communications were absent from his immediate awareness or recall. It was evident that a powerful drugging response was present at this time, so much so that I felt I was being anesthetized. This process was noted in the silences so that it seemed to be independent of speech. I experienced an instantaneous loss of sensation about my upper body/face; and a powerful urge to deflect attention, change the subject and shake off this experience by intense movement.

Using these experiences as observations, I was able to establish that the "deletions" of my interpretations of his own communications occurred just after these burst of "anesthesia." His voice would change to a drugged, slurred sound, as if he were suddenly intoxicated. He would become unable to listen and would experience an intense desire to leave the room or get off the couch, and was obviously horrified to discover that this sequence was not limited to the analytic consulting room: it occurred with his wife and colleagues, and when any intimacy was involved his capacity to attend was limited to less than thirty seconds.

In the first three years of analysis these phenomena were investigated transferentially and very little else was focused on except his capacity to listen, speak, and develop awareness of his own communication. His capacity for attention increased and with greater awareness there was increasing clarity about his inability to mean what he said or say what he meant. Thus we had a relationship in which accuracy of interpretations was severely hindered by his inability to provide me with the truth and further complicated by his not being able to listen or attend to either of us. His voice was thin and slurred much of the time and had a vibratory quality that was intensely unpleasant. When he spoke, the experience of hearing the sound was so numbing that he could not stand listening. There was a feedback loop so that by his speech in the form we came to call the use of a "number" to designate the benumbing effect, he would change state of mind almost instantly so that he was immediately out of touch and would become heavily drugged. At times he would be physically unable to move in a state similar to catatonia. This drugging effect, then, was activated by vocal sound (either his or mine at first).

Over these first three years we developed the capacity to tolerate the intense drugging interruption induced by tone, long enough for him to change his quality of sound and lighten his consciousness, like someone awakening from anesthesia. Gradually he became able to remain alert enough to attend during the entire session, which was terribly upsetting to him. Now he could suddenly hear the tonal qualities which he used elsewhere and also the sounds of others' voices, which gradually became available to him. It was the realization of his own voice and its effects, partly by comparison with others' voices now in his awareness, that led to the memory of the deadly quality of mother's voice and ushered in the return of early experiences such as her depression, constant frustration, anger, and chain-smoking. In contrast, "normal" tonality of others' voices led to sadness at the awareness of the sense of internal devastation he had experienced as a child.

His mother's voice was now heard and described as a rasping sarcasm. He recalled memories of running from it in pain as a child of two or three and isolating himself, relying on his dog, and on reading as a method of communicating virtually until his teens. He learned to hear his own voice peppered with cruel sarcasm which had the effect of inducing numbness. It seemed to me that these numbing responses, then, were related directly to painful vocal stimuli, either by feedback, in hearing his own voice, or by anticipation, in which he would drug himself before the "pain" would hit. This phenomenon is different from sleepiness in that the effect is immediate and sudden and has anesthetic qualities.

After several years his attention was keen enough to recognize the feedback effects induced by several different tones: varying from sleep, to sexual stimulation, to a sense of warmth and bliss evoked by self induced lullaby, often accompanied by pleasant imagery—all organized to interrupt the flow of our communication staying on point. These seemingly "free associations" were elaborate evasions and a form of autistic stimulation which kept him encapsulated and out of touch with me so that there was no perceived difference between my presence and absence.

Various actual melodies were used to induce states of mind. Songs were used to shift his mood and control any feeling of even momentary sadness, of which he was terrified. It was as if this patient had an internal pharmacopoeia which was utilized to produce a variety of states of mind which could be cataloged as (1) "seducers"; (2) "high-speed distractors"; (3) "numbers"; and (4) "sleepers," all of which could take the place of focused on-point communication. Each one of these states of mind involved a shift of tonal quality which became recognizable to both of us.

The analytic work took the form of a counterintelligence modality to mount and establish a rebellion against the use of these methods of distraction. At this point, anxiety became palpable for both of us and gradually broke through to his experience of rage-anxiety-frustration and grief. With the emergence of these experiences of the affect there was a sudden clear awareness of his separateness and the development of the phenomenology of two-ness in the sessions. It is possible now for him to be aware of the distracting stimuli and think through them without losing the point or getting off track. His capacity for contact has been increased by orders of magnitude, as has his capacity to learn from the experience that is increasingly available to him. His "memory" or recall problems were largely related to a lack of penetration of verbal experience in the first place, since he could not listen and could only put forward an "imitation" of human speech. He was unable to attend to incoming verbal experience as a function of his distraction and splitting, so that what appeared to be a problem of memory was related to a lack of registration of experience. I do not find these phenomena to be rare, but to occur frequently in many patients. The drugging effects can also be analogous to "excitants" and may have considerable variations from person to person.

3. Psychological Effects of Sound Density, Intonation, and Rhythm

Among the important qualities that the composer must consider is the "density" of sound. I use this term to denote a spatial quality in the listener's experience. Too great a density of sound—from too many notes, too much volume or speed—decreases interest, attentiveness and sensitivity in both player and listener. As a matter of aesthetics, it is well known that one version of tasteful improvisational playing involves sparseness which allows for spatial consideration in the receiver. Miles Davis and Ahmad Jamal are masters of this technique, which has the effect of producing an anticipatory quality. Building upon this basic rule for initiating a solo, one begins to suggest a theme which leaves room for further elaboration, and in ensemble playing includes respect for the other players who are invited to join in by virtue of the space left for them. These qualities are so well known in certain forms of Indian improvisational music that rhythmic forms on the drums produce specific spatial visual effects on the listener: codified as circles, rectangles and diamond shapes (Sambamoorthy, 1975).

With these thoughts about sound density, intonation and rhythm in mind, I would like to apply these considerations to psychoanalytic listening and present an example which is very common in everyday life as well as in one's own practice. The example has to do with the "interpretation of pain and the effect of this interpretation on the listener."

A 28-year-old pregnant woman in her second trimester was saying: "I can't stand it." [Pause.] "I can't stand it." [Pause.] "I can't stand it." [Pause.] "I can't breathe." [Pause.] "I can't breathe." [Pause.] "I can't breathe." [Pause.]—all in a very definitive, plaintive, pressured, desperate voice. My interpretation disagreed with her in that I said quietly and calmly: "No, what you mean is your breathing is more difficult." She became quiet temporarily and said: "I feel guilty." I asked her what she meant. She said:

> I just heard X [her own name] saying: "*How could* you feel that!?" and the feeling is generated from that insulting tone of voice. Then I think I'm a lousy person because I'm not enjoying being pregnant but that *doesn't mean* that I'm not enjoying being pregnant . . . My instant interpretation is that I am terrible because I cannot deal with gas pains. Then I hear: "Well, if you can't deal with gas pains, how are you going to deal with labor!?"

I have found that there is a profound difference between this "instant interpretation" which impels to immediate action and a later-arriving interpretation which is less urgent, demanding, precipitate and peremptory. This "first interpretation" is often quite autocratic, cruel and insulting, coming through with a great deal of pressure and brooking no disagreement. There is frequently a tone of contempt and violent threat associated as well, suggesting that putting forward any other point of view is not only foolhardy but dangerous because "*it is the way it is and that's that.*" The second thought emerging is more reasonable, much less pressured and allows for discussion.

These "first thoughts" were the "orders" which the patient heard for years, and it took five years of work together to develop the capacity to dissect the "first" and "second" voices from each other, as demonstrated in this example. The primary means of discovery has been to become aware of "tone" and make it clear to the patient until such time as the patient's skill in listening develops to the point of recognizing the difference between the two forms of communication and being able to tolerate the pain of the experience of the "first voice" (cruel conscience) in its unprojected form without losing consciousness or numbing to the point of loss of awareness. At that time, "second thought" has a chance of emerging and can be compared to "first thought" for discriminatory self-analytic purposes, making the distinction between the kind of "analyst" associated with the "first" and with the "second" form of thought.

I use the term "analyst" because the first voice makes "interpretations" to the patient which are directions, orders, insults, discouragements and are organized to produce a rapid response—one of immediate reactive "control," although at this point in the discussion I wish to leave the form of action blank. In this way, we can note the nature of the "analyst" with whom we are being confused. The self-interpretative process has gone on long before we have arrived on the scene and will obviously go on during and after the analysis; thus the understanding and modification of the effects of this self-interpretative process are essential for continued growth and development.

The development of the capacity to listen, especially to "musical" elements, meets with intense resistance in direct relation to the intensity of the mental pain which develops when the intonational elements register on the listener's mind. There is a pattern: an awareness of the pain in relation to the tonal elements (that is, in relation to the cruel voice) can be noted before there is any emergence of a "second" thought of alternative. Thus there is a considerable period of time in which the analysand is increasingly aware of an alarmingly rapid increase in the intensity of mental pain, with the associated diminution of defenses against it. This combination of elements produces considerable alarm and multiple retreats to the previous methodology of ablating listening and subsequent discrimination until such routes are no longer available. This lack of available defense predictably produces considerable hostility and fear of having gone too far, accompanied by a desire to end the work precipitously. It is therefore technically important to develop a simultaneous awareness of positive elements of discrimination in the sensory world, since so much of the discovery process is painful.

In this situation, the "sarcastic," demanding, hostile, insulting, interpretative first voice attacks the connection with thinking and takes over so that only its "interpretation" is left, without any correcting view from thinking. Thinking has been knocked out, leaving a dominance of pure feeling generated by the cruel "first-voice" interpretation, which is now completely dissociated from the experience. This is a kind of feedback that could be considered as a form of autohypnosis. The cruel first voice can be loud, repetitive, instantaneous, piercing, sarcastic, percussive; and it generates a painful set of feelings with great reproducibility. As one can imagine, these phenomena are not tare. It is a profound problem of psychoanalytic technique to differentiate these first-voice "interpretations" with which the patient comes already supplied and which do not constitute thinking or true interpretation at all, but are quite destructive and easily confused with the interpretations of the analyst.

I will not deal here with this discrimination, but only with the consistency of the sound elements present in the "cruel voice" so that it can be clearly heard and differentiated. Only then can any true, utilizable analytic work he instigated. This cruel first voice has a stereotyped recognizable quality which is specific to each patient in both stress (emphasis) and intonation, and would require a pitch-extraction contour to demonstrate the physical elements of its "sound" qualities in terms of melodic contour, attack, intensity, duration, and so on. Usually, before this differentiation is made, the analyst is experienced as another cruel voice which one would do better to avoid. This voice is rather like a specific drug which turns off thinking and has a defined, dosed, pharmacological effect which is quite precise.

Borrowing from the applied science of pharmacology, there are important parallels between what is considered an effective "drug" and a vocal or sound communication which has a defined effect. In the definition of the "good neuropharmacological agent," several factors have to be present. Initially, the drug must reach the site of action, presumably the brain, by crossing the blood-brain barrier. Then, there must be rapid and adequate penetration to the tissue itself by appropriate solubility and subsequent attachment to its specific site of action. Thereafter, the drug must be effectively "cleared" from the region and adapted for removal or excretion so that there is a specific, rapid turn-on-off effect for the phenomenon in question. These qualities are ideal and actually very difficult to achieve in a drug-tissue interaction.

Consider *Cannabis sativa*, for example, which takes fifteen days to clear from the central nervous system after a single dose (Lemberger, Axelrod, and Kopin, 1972), in contrast to alcohol's very rapid absorption and clearance. When we studied the metabolism of phenylethylamines in the late 1960s, there was suddenly a startling discovery: that the brain had all the equipment for producing n,n-dimethyltryptamine, a potent hallucinogen, which set investigators scrambling for ten years trying to establish psychosis as an endogenous chemical event. These ideas prepared me for the observations one can make in patients in whom these intonational prosodic "drugs" fulfill many of the neuropharmacological criteria outlined above, and in a far superior manner. The rate of onset is virtually instantaneous, the dose is controlled delicately and the effect is very specific. Furthermore, the half-life of the specific effect is very short unless the dose is repeated. I have briefly mentioned "numbers, high-speed distractors, seducers" above. I drew attention to the analogy of the specific sound effects, as also defined by musical principles. I am referring to these specific effects when I use the term mental "drug."

In using the term "drug" I am making use of an analogic imaginative conjecture and do not mean to state that there is a direct chemical effect of an intonational or prosodic sequence on the mind. Pornography is another very clear example; this time of the use of dosed, specific, repetitive, very simple fantasies which are stereotyped and produce an erectile response. This response has nothing to do with thinking but rather is experienced as a concrete reaction in which impulse goes straight to deed (Freud, 1911). Very specific organizations of fantasy are the "standards," borrowing a term from popular music, which seem to have durability and quite clear effects. One fantasy equals one direct erectile response. This clearly is a very simple model but would qualify for what Bion (1955) referred to as "speech as a form of action" in his article "Language and the schizophrenic." What I am attempting to do here is extend that aspect of language or speech as a form of action to include a variety of specific forms produced by mental drugs—that is, verbal and/or sound organizations—so that by our increasing observations as a psychoanalytic group we can establish the rules for the effects of these "communications."

We can postulate that mental "drugging" has effects on the regulation of mental pain associated with disharmonious relations to mother. Soothing effects on mental pain may be predominant here with respect to maternal vocal patterns acting on the infant's state of mind. However, other effects such as engagement and alerting processes can be recognized.

I have considered only very simple mental effects involving direct linkage between intonation and state of mind. However, this it clearly not so simple, even in popular musical forms built on defined tonal patterns. In most "standards" the tonal pattern is II, V, 1, which cycles through the structure of the song. Usually the II chord is a minor seventh, the V chord a dominant seventh and the I chord a major seventh. For example, in the key of C, II would be D minor seventh, V a G dominant seventh and I or the tonic a C major seventh.

This, then, is a series of relations called "changes," recognizable in jazz terminology, which hold through the cycle of all twelve keys. This form produces a mental "set" which has a recognizable "feel." It is likely that there are prosodic "changes" recognizable in human vocal patterns. which are effective in producing reproducible mental effects. The pattern of emotional experience in moving through the II, V, I cycle has consistency and a dramatic effect which is emphasized by changing the distribution pattern of the notes in the sequence. II minor seventh with a flatted fifth would produce a different experience in the listener, not articulable except in poetic form and beyond my capacities as a writer.

In the development of language imitation, the infant "discovers" the pain-reducing features of sound, cooing, and so on, and the effects on mental regulation by sound thereby appear in earliest infancy (some studies have indicated that these effects occur in utero [Eisenberg, 1976]). The route by which a baby could develop a dominance of autism versus autoregulation is very narrow and depends on the relations between maternal capacity and constitutional differences in the infant, determining whether the pain associated with the lack of a regulating object can be tolerated. Separation from the regulating object involves the development of object-relatedness, with reliance on self-regulatory pain decreasing uses of sound as a partial process.

In infants with a low pain threshold—through either lack of an effective maternal holding environment or constitutional differences—there is a shift in balance towards the development of autistic mechanisms which lack the flexibility or adaptive range of autoregulatory mechanisms. Here, intonational patterning is crucial because it is among the earliest of all means of communication which establish contact with the world of external objects and the self. Meaning, then, is often displaced in dominance from a symbolic verbal world to a tonal world in which the symbolic content is virtually secondary or diminished in importance. This can result in verbal communication being developed for other uses exclusive of external communication and hidden from ordinary awareness, so that conversation is not orientated towards communicating specific symbolic meaning to the outside, but is a feedback autistic selfstimulatory mode organized to produce a specific mind set utilized to prevent any awareness of separation from the object.

One of the problematic features of psychoanalysis has been its primary focus on psychopathology rather than a more balanced approach to developmental processes. If we can study the means by which communication is obstructed in the transference, then we can also find the means by which it is facilitated. The notion of "an internal pharmacopoeia" can have a purely pathological prejudice, but I think it needs to be considered on a much broader basis. What about mental mood elevators and euphoriants. to which we could do a serious disservice simply by calling them manic defenses? How can verbal communication be used as an analogy to musical accompaniment? Perhaps vocal mirroring or echoing are appropriate forms to be considered in future studies as analytic "accompaniment"—not only in terms of verbal content with which analysts are familiar, such as using the patient's language forms, but also with regard to intonational patterns, emphasis, rhythm and pause structure.

For example, if the analyst is speaking slowly and deliberately to a patient whose own speech is built on a rapid rhythm, and it is clear to the analyst that the patient is not listening, often the patient becomes impatient, is unable to restrain the flow of speech, and may interrupt the analyst. If the analyst continues his interpretation *while* being interrupted it becomes clear to the patient that he is interrupting and he may not remember what the analyst is saying, partly because the analytic communication is being broken up by the patient and partly because the two are speaking at the same time.

The analyst may be able to show the process in action to the patient: that he does not take in the analyst's communications because he is not listening but rather talking at the same time. Frequently the patient will ask for the analyst to repeat the communication. If the analyst does, he may give the patient the "illusion" of repeating, but he actually cannot "repeat" because the context has changed. Drawing attention to this point may produce angry frustration, but complying with the patient's wish furthers the illusion that what has been missed can be repeated. This form of "accompaniment" can be disharmonious but may be very useful. Operating at the same rhythm as the patient under these conditions may be quite agreeable to the patient but not suitable to establishing the conditions for learning from experience. Here the analyst must be sensitive to the rhythm of interactional communication that can facilitate verbal digestion. Rhythm of speech can also be too slow for appropriate linkage to be made. Note that I am giving only a simple particular example of a general issue.

Herbert Rosenfeld has made practical references to the tempo of speech in relation to the capacity to apprehend meaning. When one interprets the effect of excessive velocity of communication, one may use an interpretation phrased in ordinary conversational tempo, but what is this tempo? Is ordinary tempo a reference point for the efficacy of reception and registration of verbal thought according to metronomic accuracy? One would like to think that there are broad generalizations of tempo between individuals which would suit as a standard for a range which would allow for both affective and ideational reception.

Velocity may be used as a means of avoiding the experience of painful affect, and the ideational representative may get across diminished in meaning, because of its emptiness of affective load. The analysis of a variety of forms of mental pain may yield understanding of a pressure of experience that leads to increased velocity of speech. Painful mental experiences that are concrete and persecutory can lead to reflexive attempts to evacuate them in phantasy, leading to increased speed or velocity. The analysis of such experience often leads to effective slowing, and is an extremely important mode *of* operational interpretation. A form of interpretation such as "when you speak so quickly, you find it difficult to understand me" may allow the emergence of feeling and an effective registration of mental experience so that the feelings can be integrated with the thought content.

Socrates considered himself a kind of mental midwife assisting in the birth of others' ideas. We know something of the method of inquiry he was reputed to use in Plato's dialogues. His accompaniment stimulated the development of others' growth. Accompaniment in modern improvisational music is initially a cushion for the soloist. The rhythm must he rock-solid, and suggested methods of accompaniment involve intense listening for the direction of the soloist so that support can be provided, whether melodically or by chordal fills, depending on the skill of the accompanist. Among musicians, this skill is highly regarded as one of the most necessary and difficult tasks in playing; yet it is virtually unnoticed by the audience, who are moved by the soloist's capacity for extension and virtuosity.

What is its conversational equivalent? Are there analytic interventions as forms of action which are the equivalents of sophisticated musical accompaniment? What are the considerations which involve timing these interventions so that they are precise and facilitating background experiences that make it more possible for patients to develop their explorative capacities? What are the appropriate intonations for these interpretations? When, for example, can one use imitative intonation (imitating the rhythm of the patient) to demonstrate obstructive prosodic mechanisms without being experienced as cruelly mocking? By obstructive prosodic mechanisms I mean the use of the combination of pitch, vocal quality, emphasis or lack of it, which have a feedback effect on the speaker or the listener of shutting down the function of attention, and practical purposes of closing the mind. A simple example would involve the employment of a prosecuting tone in asking a question which would induce defense and closure versus the use of a genuine inquiry which would lend itself to curiosity and exploration.

If we begin to make these observations, we can then begin to develop a musical ear for vocal processes in ourselves and develop a notation system for recording these observations more precisely so that we can bring these infraverbal experiences into analytic investigations and stimulate the patient's capacity for listening, which is an essential feature for the development of any sophisticated verbal interactive process.

The musical notation system, although very precise, still leaves considerable room for varying interpretation when what is written is played accurately. The communication of the feel of a series of dotted eighth notes is very different for the classical player from what it is to the jazz musician. The notes are written exactly alike but are interpreted very differently. Many classically trained musicians with excellent technique cannot intuit the jazz "feel." Even with a good psychoanalytic notation system we will expect difficulties of this sort, but the gap between the experience in the session and the reporting of it would probably be diminished. An increased psychoanalytic awareness of the musical (nonverbal) aspects of vocal communication would develop.

Psychoanalysis would then be in a position to make important contributions in assessing the quality and prominence of vocal communication and could carry research into areas beyond behaviorism, such as the study of propaganda. The induction of specific affects by the subtle devices of mass-communication media is of serious social concern: not only the loss of meaning and sincerity but also the decreasing ability of the audience to recognize sincerity.

Chapter 9

On the Imitation of Human Speech

An exploration of the distortion and misuse of verbal communication is developed with special reference to the imitation of human speech. The problems associated with the thinning and lysis of an encapsulated autistic state are considered with emphasis on the discovery of painful affects. The process of the communication associated with living-in-a-capsule and speaking as though true symbolic communication was occurring with the analyst is considered. The transformation from this primitive state to a state of mind in which sincere authentic communication is possible is discussed. Clinical material is presented to show some of the difficulties involved in the disordered thinking that leads to imitation speech. Special emphasis is placed on the use of an induced fixed state of mind which can take many forms. These inducers organize a "time arrested" phantasied state related to a prenatal phantasy and are used as a part of the barrier to contact with reality.

The Appearance of the Autistic Barrier

I want to describe a series of structures which can have infinite variation yet have constantly conjoined qualities. In so doing, I wish to set out the main points of this communication that will be fleshed out subsequently:

1. There can be a barrier which separates the patient from true contact with the analyst. This barrier is maintained rigidly although it is subtle.

2. The patient does not engage in true object relations but appears to. The difference between true and false contact can be observed through qualities of the patient's speech. Speech is used as a form of

action. Sensation rather than meaning is achieved. Speech is used concretely.

3. A barrier to contact disguises an hallucinatory world born of intolerance to frustration. These hallucinatory images have a fixed quality or stereotypy which determines the patient's emotional state. I liken these fixed fantasy states to virtual reality and call them virtual fantasies. They are usually known by the patient and are carefully protected as they offer a sense of security, safety from uncertainty, and a belief in "self-control."

4. When the analyst's interpretations fail to reify the image the patient has in mind, a barrier is erected by the patient. The interpretations are stopped by the barrier and transformed to sensation rather than meaning.

5. Lysis of the barrier results in extreme disorientation while "orientation" means the presence of the system of virtual fantasies remaining in place.

6. When the barrier is breached, certain changes occur similar to the emergence from a prenatal state. Dizziness, the sensation of cold, disorientation, and sensations of extreme pressure attend the lysis of the barrier. These phenomena are linked to phantasies associated with birth.

7. When these disturbing emotions can be tolerated, growth can occur. The barrier to input from the external world is opened when the pain associated with the lysis of the barrier can be understood without automatic withdrawal.

8. I am using the notion of imitative speech to refer to something which sounds like speech but is not communicating symbolic meaning. Rather this form of speech is used to maintain the barrier just described and to induce replicable hallucinatory fantasies.

Much has been discussed recently about autism, from descriptions of the "phenomena in children" to the recognition that there is such an entity in adults. The confusional versus encapsulated forms have been differentiated and described by Frances Tustin (1981), and a less well-known post obsessional subclinical form has been described by Donald Meltzer and his co-workers (1975).

In an earlier chapter (see Chapter 4) I described some of the clinical findings related to the difficulties encountered in the recognition of imitative speech, or mimesis, in that the imitation in these individuals is an imitation of human speech itself. The problem emerges when one attempts an interpretive intervention using articulate speech and attempts to address the interpretation to a precise point and finds that the analysand is speaking a different language, one which has at its base an action component rather than a symbolic meaning.

From the analysand's unconscious point of reference, the problem involves giving a response which "seems" like the real thing so that the incoming interpretation can be intercepted before registration. This blockade maintains the phantasy of the hermetic seal or encapsulated barrier. This maneuver is meant to give the listener the impression of a satisfactory response. Upon further investigation, the analyst finds that there is no change, only seeming cooperation. So far, all of these considerations are familiar.

In the encapsulated autism described by Tustin (1981) and Meltzer (1975), there has been a cursory discussion of the lack of development of symbolic language. Bion (1955, 1970) described the use of language in psychotic patients as a form of action bypassing meaning. He postulated that the formation of language was integrally related to the establishment of the depressive position. Whole object relations are hindered in relation to the deficit in the development and use of symbolic language. In this article, I explore adult patients who fit the description of Meltzer's subclinical autism and who utilize language as a form of action leading to a failure in development.

In "Language and the Schizophrenic" (1955), Bion sketches the stages of recognition of psychotic states in reference to the use of language. He further elaborates the effects of the "meaningless" but action-oriented communication in *Attention and Interpretation* (Bion, 1970). The practical problem there is the following.

A. The patient behaves as though he were in an encapsulated state with a semipermeable barrier interposed between the outside world and himself.

B. Both the analyst and analysand are using articulate speech differently, the analyst to communicate meaning, that is to say using language having precise reference in which the words and phrases refer specifically to something. The analysand must block the contact, recognizing the "intent" to communicate, by the analyst's incoming language, which to him means to penetrate the barrier and either stop or change the experience.

C. The patient, as Bion (1970) reminds us, mistakes feeling pain for suffering it. Frustration and intense pain are equated. Pain is sexualized and thereby experienced as inflicted or accepted but not suffered—no meaning develops and a failure of mental growth occurs. Learning is confused with increasing skill at recognizing incoming experience soon enough to deflect it.

D. This experience of the deflected communication is often very sensuous and intense and repeated endlessly as the contact may produce intense sensations which can be sexualized.

E. In Bion's (1970) model, the patient feels the pain of an absence of fulfillment of his desires (to have whatever he has in mind). The absent fulfillment is experienced as a no-thing, and the emotion aroused by the no-thing is felt as indistinguishable from the no-thing. The emotion is, replaced by a no-emotion. Bion (1970) continues, "In practice, this can mean no feeling at all or an emotion such as rage which is a Column 2 emotion, that is an emotion of which the fundamental function is denial of another emotion. As a Column 2 element, all felt emotion is a no-emotion In this respect, it is analogous to 'past' or future as representing the 'place' where the present used to be before all time was annihilated. The place where time was (or feeling was or a no-thing of any kind was) is then similarly annihilated." He continues, "Some patients with which I am familiar achieve a state to which I wish to apply the term non-existence" (p. 20).

F. In Bion's (1970) model, the patient has annihilated time, meaning, symbolic articulate speech and linking associated with violent destructiveness as a function of envy of life itself (presumably in the analyst). There is the destruction of "reality" replaced with the mental detritus resulting from the destruction. Subsequent envy of the life that the object can have becomes a result of the frustration or failure to meet his desires. This summary serves to indicate the state of mind of the patient in order to describe the nature of the receptor to which articulate speech is to be addressed.

Following the abstraction of these desires of the patient for instantaneous reification, there is a wish to be without speech or need for communication. In specific, the patient may say in response to interpretation, "That's not what I had in mind." Further examination reveals a complex set of images (visual or otherwise) which the patient expects to make real by the utterance of the "precise interpretation" which can never approximate to what they have in mind. The expectation by the analysand is that the verbal productions of the analyst will reify in perpetuity the deeply held phantasy/expectation carried in mind by the analysand. The certainty of frustration and failure of the analyst to produce this long expected result leads to demeaning hostility and despair. Language has been expected to have a result involving reification as a fulfillment of the patient's desires. In Bion's example, the patient has established limited contact with the analyst and is furious because his delusions or hallucinations are not reified. My patient has not achieved this realization, although he suspects it to be true. Bion (1970) formulates,

> The patient then may be seen as facing a choice; either he may allow his intolerance of frustration to use what might be otherwise a no-thing to become a thought, and so achieve the freedom that Freud (1911) describes or he might use what might be a no-thing as the foundation for a system of hallucinosis (p. 17).

Bion (1970) continued,

> The word "dog" represents different realizations in scientific inquiry and hallucinosis; but the word "dog" is itself not the same when it is representing a realization in scientific inquiry and an element belonging to the domain of hallucinatory transformations. It is sometimes useful to regard it as analogous to the visual image in a reversible transformation. In the visual image, the marks of a drawing on paper remain unchanged but mean two faces or a vase; similarly, dog may mean dog or god. Hallucinations are not representations. They are things in themselves born of intolerance of frustration and desire (p. 18).

What happens when desire and fulfillment are the same and the patient lives in a state of mind which one could call hallucinosis which is used as a fixed regulator blockading the input to the mind? The phantasy of the "seal" is retained but in the state of hallucinosis to which I refer, there is psychoanalytic verbal "intercourse" which retains seemingly smooth interaction to response. The elaboration of speech, prepared dreams and especially prepared material as "problems to discuss" maintain the decoying system so that it appears that a conversation is going on. These practiced maneuvers maintain the "dream-hallucination" unless the psychoanalyst's interpretations reach close to the mark. The patient's rejoinder is frequently, "That isn't what I had in mind." At first, this seemed to me to be a remarkably omniscient expectation and usually was associated with hostility. One finds that the response is literal and refers accurately to the fact that the interpretation is not what is held in mind. "I don't see what you mean" as a response often refers to the failure of the interpretation to yield an image which can be compared to the image the patient has in mind. One can compare the response of a patient who receives the same interpretation and associates to it in context evolving further developed material accessing levels of mind previously unexplored. The patient I am describing now engages in a variety of splitting or distancing maneuvers.

The patient behaves as though the analyst "should be" fused with him. Then he would achieve the match expected, but words ought not to be necessary. The use of language or words indicates space between individuals which must be negotiated. Language is felt to involve grave inadequacies at all times. With the "failure to achieve fusion," the analysand must then keep distance from emotional contact since separateness is hated. This process of quiet hatred and disappointment occurs with the avoidance of contact unnoticed and unsaid by both analyst and analysand. Only when this phenomenon becomes the subject of the analytic interaction do overt defensive maneuvers become evident.

One very subtle defense is the use of a particular sense to divide the attention. While the patient is associating and I am interpreting, he is following the outlines of a door, ceiling tiles, or tracing the pattern of a plant leaf or branch with his eyes. One can feel the thinness of the interaction at that time which aids in interpretation. He is "safe"—no contact or diminished contact has been achieved. If the barrier is discovered and the choice can be made to tolerate the frustration-pain, a sudden change can be observed. Initially, intense emotions including anxiety and sadness can be noted. These emotions can be immediately blocked by a drugging stupor communicable to analyst and analysand both. With persistent interpretation over time, frustration can be tolerated better and yields a new configuration which the patient refers to as disorienting. "Orientation" turns out to be "the addiction to the previously held mind-set organized by a particular phantasy." I analogize the hermetically sealed "oriented closed" prior state of mind to a form of autism in which a timeless state is maintained by a fixed phantasy structure. I am remaining deliberately abstract as in my experience the variations of these fixed orienting phantasies are numerous. These phantasies can be borrowed from the culture or internally evolved and are used as a virtual world, quite complex yet predictable. There can be infinite variation in form. The use to which these phantasies are put, then, are to prevent frustration and the experience of loss while maintaining a strong emotional tone "played" by the phantasy by induction. This consistent emotional tone then constitutes the reassuring belief that everything is the same. No change is felt to have occurred except when it is ineluctably obvious. This emotional tone is played to the external world, then, and appears as though it is direct and real.

The following is a clinical example involving what I refer to as a virtual fantasy taken from the ninth year of the analysis of a 42-year-old male mathematician.

Clinical Example

The patient enters, eyes averted, and shoots a quick, glaring glance toward me. I immediately have a momentary suspicion that he is deliberately "up to something." He lies on the couch with a smooth athletic motion. I gradually begin to get a headache and feel numb at the same time. There is a recognizable deterioration in the clarity of my state of mind and suddenly I notice a sense of emotional thinness. The patient states, "I don't know what to say." I interpret that he has been attempting to get rid of me by producing pain in me so I will leave him alone. He agrees and I can feel a change in his attention which intensifies. I have a phantasy that something is about to "happen." As I feel my attention increasing and the pain remit, he begins to cry, which is a very different pattern. He then begins to undergo clonic twitching including arms, legs and torso in short bursts. This goes on for quite a time. These motions are quite exaggerated while at the same time I have the impression he is attempting either to hide this phenomenon or downplay it. The crying continues with a muffled quality. I interpret, "I think you are seeing something that you feel is very upsetting from which you are attempting to split you and me away from at the same time." The clonic twitching increases and the sobbing intensifies to sickening sounds of extreme pain. I interpret, "You are purposely producing an image which you can hold in mind to induce a specific set of feelings that you can use to avoid any contact with me." There is a silence and a profound sense that the patient has mentally disappeared. He agrees and states that he has been observing a large series of people being strapped into serial electric chairs and electrocuted at once.

This is not the first time this image has been used, and has been part of a script this patient has been developing for a film. He then describes the scene with the same sense of divided attention. I notice an intensifying headache again and a desire to leave the room myself. I interpret as I have had many episodes of this sort of thing, that he feels superior in being able to maintain his images which are by now far more real than anything I might say to him. He agrees. The awareness of a barrier existing between us is quite clear to both of us. His responses do not extend what I interpret but serve to keep me at a considerable distance. This same patient has a variety of similar fantasies which can produce sexual sensations or tears or extreme emotional tension on cue, rather like a "method" actor who can depend on the production of feelings at will by changing the internal image. The patient expresses a predilection for crying and states that he not only feels relief but also enjoys the sensation. He can say this not in direct response to a point-on-point interpretation but only after considerable evidence that he feels I have been sufficiently distanced. We have learned subsequently in the analytic work these emotional tricks were consciously utilized to keep his mother at bay, who is both psychotic (hospitalized for periods of time), had shock treatments, and could be both physically and sexually invasive with him. Space does not permit further elaboration of these dynamics here. I present this example as a means of demonstrating the barrier to contact, the use of imagery, which in this situation appears to be consciously induced although subsequently, years later in the analysis, has been found to be a significant part of a negative maternal transference.

Psychoanalytic Tactics Relating to the Breakdown of the Barrier

In this discussion, I wish to describe some problems in the switch from "virtual reality" to object relations. This emergence is painful and is connected to a series of constantly conjoined phenomena which have a relation to the birth process, especially labor. Disorientation, dizziness, vertigo, and sudden cold associated with intense dread occur when an interpretation is so close that it penetrates and is felt as an intrusion (Paul, 1981; see Chapter 4). Continued progress leads to more frequent contact, usually hated, in the psychoanalytic sessions with no further reference to outside life being made. Later, one may find that a considerable improvement in the patient's outside life occurs.

Certain consistent problems are related within the group of patients who operate behind an "autistic" barrier. The strategy of a psychoanalytic approach, then, must take up the problems associated with the mental journey beyond this barrier. I shall briefly list them and subsequently elaborate more fully. In the psychoanalytic process, one task is establishing contact with external reality. This process involves movement from the addictive standard, time arresting virtual world in which a barrier exists to "protect" the individual from pain, frustration, and a panoply of other emotions including sadness, loss, disorientation, and uncertainty. The virtual organizing phantasy structures, including autostimulation, the forms of which can be infinite, provide a consistent, organized, and ordered world of feeling which is used by the patient as an attempt to establish meaning but results in a lack of it. The painful discovery that one's emotions are not to be trusted to reflect the experience of reality can be most disturbing. The use of feeling as an instrument of establishing meaning must be retooled. With each step away from certain virtual, established experience, painful affect evolves as previously stated. The autistic barrier "protects" the time arresting virtual phantasy which produces reassuring belief that no change can occur. The effect of establishing a breach in the barrier results in experiences similar to the labor process and emergence from a prenatal state. The "disorientation" described indicates movement away from the "security" of this prenatal state.

In the analytic work, care must be taken to detail the understanding of the anatomy of this virtual world. The components of the virtual phantasy structure need consistent, repeatable, immediate elaboration in order to "work." Establishing the morphology and function of these phantasies is met with intense resistance from archaic superego sources as previously described (Paul, 1989; see Chapter 8). This resistance is in the service of the maintenance of the barrier. As this to and fro of foray out of capsular mental life to uncertainty and painful disorientation can be allowed, there develops a gradual understanding of stereotypic attack blockade from primitive superego sources. The analysand not only gains confidence based on understanding but becomes a collaborator with the analyst when the price of the maintenance of this virtual world is recognized and gradually worked through. The demonstration that the virtual world produces exciting sensation rather than meaning is crucial to the work. Otherwise, the pull to mental masturbatory phantasies as a way of life is too great to tolerate the grief which occurs when the time arresting function is less active. As a psychoanalyst, one has the problem of the analysand's deeply held belief that their virtual experience is the "truth." One problem is that interpretations by the patient emerging from archaic internal sources carry the belief that the only escape from the depression induced by the cruel mutilation of the personality has only been "cured" or substituted for by the deployment of this virtual world. The patient fears being left with nothing. This repetition pattern maintains a profound immaturity and incapacity for the toleration of pain and frustration and subsequently leads to continued reliance on autostimulatory mechanisms.

The reader will recognize the instrumental quality of the logic employed by the analysand. Inhibition of the deployment of the virtual world leads to severe emotional pain. Therefore, "*stop everything*" becomes the paradigm for "control" or being in control. Further reactivation of the virtual phantasy occurs with relief from the certain pain resulting from allowing frustration to form the basis of thought. The patient believes that the pain resulting from the restraint leading to thought is the cause of pain. Change in this mechanism threatens the individual's belief in their sanity and is experienced as hurling them into chaos. Thinking is felt to lead to catastrophic experience and is experienced "correctly" as the disorganizing process. The organization which is altered by thinking is the virtual phantasy linked to encapsulation.

The process of development from maintenance of the transmission of psychic experience with the virtual (as if) phantasy in place to contact with the outside directly is exceedingly slow. Paradoxically, change when experienced is very rapid but cannot be tolerated and leads to an abrupt interruption and breakdown of communication with reintroduction of extreme concretism (puns, literal interpretations of obviously complex experience, sometimes quite violently). There are similarities to the negative therapeutic reaction which may mimic envy or extreme hostility, but this attack is employed to stop the communication and the attendant severe anxiety initiated by contact.

Gradually the analysand begins to tolerate the sadness, depression, and intense, psychic pain which I believe is very primitive, perhaps like the experience of a "load" of current being passed through too small a conductor. The intensity of this "pain" can be so great as to bring forth an infantile state of pain prior to verbal thought (either a function of the deployment of the depressive position or the very earliest pain prior to verbal thought). The point I wish to emphasize is that the patient's conscious cooperation in not employing the conscious elements of the virtual addictive phantasy leads to this extremely painful state of affairs. Continuing the analytic process requires a very deep trust in the analyst's capacity to tolerate and suffer the pain benignly. At the same time the analysand has developed the ability to recognize and oppose propaganda which would have automatically established the blockade leading to the maintenance of the phantasy. This complex form of cooperation can only be approached when F (Faith) (Bion, 1970) is strengthened enough to allow for the exposure.

During the time the addictive virtual phantasy is in place, there is a "bottom," a limiting barrier to these painful experiences and communication goes on in a smooth, nondepressed, often quite seemingly interesting but meaningless way. This provides the pleasant, sensuous interchange that can be enjoyable to both analyst and analysand. Typically, the intonation carries the experience in a similar way such that one can note the feeling of importance or perhaps purpose in what appears to sound confident and may indeed be confident as far as the analysand is concerned. Care must be maintained vigilantly that this same pseudo confidence is not engaged in by the analyst, no matter how tempting. One can see that as the length of time increases that the patient can tolerate life without the addictive phantasy, there is always regret that the old ways gradually lose their appeal. Not only is the pain and depression often intense, but many affects emerge that are experienced as foreign, unknown, strange, and in combinations that have no previous meaning or experience. There is loss of what is perceived as a familiar self on which the analysand has come to depend. There is fear of the vulnerability to experience from the outside which now registers in producing contact with a truer "read" of what is occurring in the external environment. The patient could not have paid "emotional mind" to the experience previously. As a result, "odd" experiences arise; the world that has been fixed in the mind of the analysand by their own design now yields a different experience, usually surprising and not always pleasant. Frequently, those who have been thought to have been friends (by idealization) seem different and yet, upon reflection, there is the increasingly sad realization that one has simply avoided what one knew but dismissed. By contrast, there may be the opposite experience that those who have been maligned may turn out to have been friends. Gratitude is not possible in individuals who have this barrier, as acknowledgment of any external contact is too disorienting. "Orientation" describes a reference to the previous link to the virtual addictive phantasy. Gratitude requires the ability to experience something coming into the self from the outside especially in relation to an object.

The Use of Simulation

I do not wish to exclude everyday phenomena from orientation to these virtual phantasies. A man buys a computer program to use at home along with a chair that changes attitude, pitch, and yaw, which accompanies visual imagery on a screen simulating the experience of flying a jet fighter. One sees the instruments in the cockpit and, by computerized shifts in the visual display, there are reproducible images generated. These images lead to a mental state in which the sensations, images, and feelings evoked correspond to "slipping into the wind" in an A-10 fighter, simulating each exact step in the landing of the fighter on a moving aircraft carrier. One becomes accustomed to the experience with which the program acquaints one and develops a skill in mastering the configuration of elements necessary to the control of the aircraft during a variety of complex situations which are close enough to real experience as to be of value in training for the real event. One develops skill in maneuvering the virtual aircraft under a variety of circumstances including emergencies which can be programmed to be used in developing experience which would not be available in any other way. This example is a constructive use of a virtual world which reproduces complex mental experiences organized in patterns which gradually achieve familiarity with increasing experience.

Suppose while you are conducting a psychoanalytic session with such a trained individual, you find that they are landing their A-10 Hornet on the deck of a carrier. This subject was not the topic of the conversation. In fact, it was about the anxiety which had occurred reaching quite intense proportions in relation to intense numbness which had arisen while driving to the appointment on the freeway. The numbness and drugged sensation had been so powerful as to raise questions as to the wisdom of pulling off the road and returning home. Only considerable previous experience with this phenomenon has allowed him to understand the organization of this deadened state of mind to cope with the mental pain associated with the emerging feelings under consideration. He knows his intense rage which he has been able to keep to himself was a function of suppression of his frustration and pain at experiencing the penetration of others' painful feeling states. He was at his limit in being able to tolerate them. Being afraid that the analytic contact would lead to greater intensity of feeling, he was able to intercept his ingrained, drugging defense in order to arrive on time to the session. Alternating between oblique, superficial contact and an acknowledgment of his mental state of affairs, I was able to notice and question slight movements of his eyes and body position revealing the various repeated aspects of his simulation of the landing process on a virtual aircraft carrier. This "landing" was going on behind our conversation and was used to diminish the intensity of the psychic pain. Discovery of the process of this "secret" and his realizations that my interpretations were not attacks made it possible for him to "dose" himself with the active use of the virtual phantasy to control the intensity of his extreme anxiety. He could then inform me himself about these landing phantasies elaborated by full cockpit instrument readings bringing him home to the mother ship and immediately reducing his anxiety. Separation anxiety now occurred for the first time as he found the analytic sessions essential to his understanding of his work and family relations, in which he noted similar feelings as had been previously described at the beginning of the session. At that time, he felt he needed the analysis more than the preservation of the learned virtual phantasy having discovered the effect of supervening numbness and loss of contact with both his family and work mates.

Describing the countertransference associated with my detection of a patient out of contact is challenging. The feeling of thinness which varies with one's approach is definitive. A verbal direct approach leads to an increased quality of "feeling of thinness." Excursions away from the point are usually relieving and can lead to a sense of enjoyment and safety. One often has the "sense" that one would be a lot wiser "not" to make a direct interpretation. Often there can be visually dominant language that can bring one's attention to a primary sensory mode being utilized. There can be an experience of being flooded by sensory communication. Close range or long range senses may be involved which can be used instrumentally to either distance or produce a lack of contact (Paul and Carson, 1980; see Chapter 3). If short range senses are used where long range experience would be appropriate, then one has touch, taste or smell rather than vision. In this mismatch a failure to connect is achieved. Virtual imagery in this regard is a good analogy as one has the impression of a false sense of focus when one looks at an object submerged in a pool of water. The apparent location is different than the actual location. In these individuals under description, their apparent location is different than their authentic location. This last point is a subjective impression, a general function of the countertransference and is inadequate for scientific purposes. One could raise the question, "Where is authentic location?" The response to be effective depends upon the analyst's capacity for at-one-ment with O (Bion, 1970).

I give this as a rather obvious use of a learned virtual phantasy to introduce the infinitude of forms which these phantasies can have. There can be forms of phantasy which are strictly virtual or others employing one or more internal sense derived images from memory which organize to produce a strong mental effect. This can involve the sense of security and especially reproducible "orientation" to the experience which is played in the mind to produce familiarity. I am concerned about whether or not there is a clear differentiation between what is being defined here as a virtual phantasy and the concept of internal unconscious phantasy as elaborated by Melanie Klein and Susan Isaacs (1970). What seems clear to me is that the organization by which these repeatable organized structures are transmitted to consciousness is in the service of suppression or inhibition of the emergence of a deeper, more primordial and ever more painful experience. These phantasies, in my experience, thus far dominate and organize the state of mind and lead to behaviors based on the conscious affects they induce. Their use seems to be organized as Column 2 elements (Bion, 1962) and prevent the flow of free association leading to discovery of deeper layers. The virtual fantasy that I described is stereotyped and is used as an inducer of replicable experience and is notable in that its usage becomes fixed. These fantasies are usually stimulating and produce strong images, sensations, and affects which give the sense-of-being-in a situation which is grossly different than the circumstances of reality.

One striking example of the use of a virtual phantasy was notable in a sixty-year-old male engineer whose job entailed a highly technical liaison between the Air Force and various satellite communication encryption devices from ground to space and space to space organization of operations codes. This highiy sophisticated, humorous, but very disturbed diminutive man, utilized imagery to convince himself that he was a teenage girl which required a conscious feat of imagination. His visual fantasies involved transvestism of a stereotyped teenage quality which had to change with the style. This fantasied disguise, which required secrecy, was a relief in the sense that it provided a feeling of safety and comfort and was a fixed world of phantasy, the primary organizer of which was fixed time so as to prevent getting older. The teenage girl fantasies were organized to be the opposite of being a sixty-year-old man concerned about aging and retirement. One quality of these phantasies is their involvement with sanctuary and control of the difficulties encountered by living in the real world—the trick is not to, while giving the illusion that one is. The "real" life is behind the scenes in the "simulator," however it is organized. In an earlier chapter (Paul, 1981; see Chapter 4), I described this man's concern with maintaining exact to the degree temperature regulation against drafts and air conditioning variations by wearing two to three pairs of long winter underwear. He could detect a single degree variation which produced severe anxiety and had a relation to a phantasy of being in the womb. Like a series of Chinese boxes, the teenage girl fantasy had to be analyzed before the more rigid and structured prenatal phantasies were elucidated and described. While some virtual fantasies are conscious and visual, they are often part of a deeper unconscious phantasy such as the above description.

The quality of time arresting constancy, sanctuary, and even pleasure, and a notable lack of persecutory experience is linked with a concrete rigidity and diminished use of projective identification. It is as though these individuals have been hermetically sealed and only are moved to pain when this autistic barrier is pierced. I want to emphasize the seeming normalcy of these individuals who appear "just like" others, talk "just like" others, and move "just like" whomever they imitate, "just like" or mimetic activity being the chief skill necessary to produce an effective disguise. These qualities are at least in part what I am using to differentiate these phantasies from those described by Klein and Isaacs. Often these "virtual fantasies" are preconscious. Even so, I would not like to claim them as being definitively different, but nonetheless worthy of description in their inductive role.

Imitation of Human Speech

The "control" of state of mind is inordinately complex. So far I have stressed the importance of voluntary processes directed by the individual. In addition, unconscious mental operations which can be seen to be quite elaborate may have a concrete quality similar to and/or leading to action. The example given below can be assigned a grid category, C6, (Bion, 1962) in which visual elements in a "dream" are ordered in a sequence which has a causal assumption.

In previous months prior to this dream, the patient, a forty-five-year-old man who had been clearly psychotic and was in his tenth year of psychoanalysis, had allowed a separation from his elderly psychotic parents. He had been addicted to caring for them, in substitution for leading his own life. They could be counted upon to produce powerful, disturbing influences with astonishing regularity. Suffice it to say that after exposure to either of them, he noted a severe diminution in his capacity to think and was so depressed, the psychic pain being so severe, that he took to bed, often recovering within several days. He timed these "exposures" so that the "threat" of effective external living, such as productive writing or involvement with a woman who was appropriate, could always be thwarted. In these activities, he used his parents' predictable stereotyped responses as an effective part of what could be thought of as a complex machine (Rube Goldberg) which had a defined, causal sequence. This negative response could effectively remove him from the field of external activity and maintain a time-arresting state of mind similar to his childhood during which painful sensations were created and maintained as an addiction. This orientation to an encapsulated time zone of feelings was constantly organized and re-organized in the transference.

A combination of steady work demonstrating the failure to actually arrest time showed him the delusional purpose of these activities. The thinning of the "capsule" allowed contact of a direct nature which was not only disorienting and extremely painful but allowed for work to go on in his creative writing that had a different character leading to development. Direct contact in which an interpretation was felt to penetrate showed, in that he remembered it and was able to compare the exact wording to recognize alterations he produced which previously would have slanted the meaning to harshness. This altered meaning would have been attributed to the analyst. After some years experience he was able to differentiate the distortions and "use" the interpretations to good account. This process had the unpleasant effect of demonstrating a kind of progress in the work that showed a time line in which it was clear that a gradation of ability to use the psychoanalytic work increased with years and was related to a diminution of delusional, paranoid activity. This recognition of time usually instituted a violent attack on linking, which would re-establish the sensuous, depressing affects he would produce by the establishment of a visual process, clearly leaving me out, and which was reported from his "capsule" at times in a manner that sounded as though the patient was enclosed in a large jar. In this "capsular phantasy," there could be an order re-instituted which led to sensation and not meaning, usually quite painful and communicated to me in such an intense way that it was very difficult for me to maintain contact. Sensations of numbness, deadness, and often intense depression, and a feeling that I can only describe as plowing through a thick pudding, would occur with regularity upon any registration of time by the patient. We both became familiar with these phenomena, and he began gradually and now more urgently to be concerned about the "waste of time" and the "years going by" that could not be recouped no matter how precisely he could create and recreate the same affective states.

During this latter period of progress in the analysis, he related a dream, which he had taken to writing in a detailed notebook, and reported during periods of desperation. When he "gave up" the visual fantasizing encapsulated drugged state which he could recognize as a "mental masturbation" of a kind we had often detailed and would allow a "dosed" experience of contact in which he had the partial experience of "control," he felt anxious. Again, "control" meant that he had his mental foot on the brakes and felt that he could abate the terrifying feeling of disorientation which was no longer as overwhelmingly painful as before.

I. He began, "If it isn't an action, what is it?" He then reported a dream. *I am looking at loading docks in my father's warehouse— these are long and narrow and not connected to the building. I am looking at a layer of concrete that needs to match some internal level—I see construction bolts—there is something there which needs to find a certain level to fit or something.*

II. *NASA has invented a device that blows an astronaut out of a building into a chute under air pressure leading into a cockpit. The chute does not connect—I'm worried about air turbulence flow—if the cockpit was closed it would create back pressure, so I tell my brother where the air is going (a) it came out of vents; (b) it recirculated through the engine—then I explained it to my brother. Once it's invented, now what? They don't need to invent anything else because that's how it's done from then on. They just keep repeating it. In this situation, it's where the answer is actually the death of the question.*

Then I'm seeing it from a big distance, as though I'm looking at slides —I'm seeing an image of the space shuttle—I'm bored with the images. There is a red one, one with writing on it. A crowd is cheering on O.J. Simpson. The guys there must have been around a lot—he was charming, so they liked him. That's why they wrote what they wrote.

I interpreted that he was showing me a concrete communication in which, if he could raise the level of feeling, he could be blown out of his concrete bunker into an open cockpit that he was having engineering difficulties with. He could recognize the repetition and increasing distance from contact and instead of being fascinated with his virtuosity of image production, he was bored with it since he could realize the increasing distance from contact, no matter how elaborate his visual production was, the result was still the same, distance. The patient agreed, although I wasn't positive, that his response registered true agreement, but continued with the dream, which I hadn't realized I had interrupted.

> *I'm in a car, driving away with my girl. She leans over close to the guy next to her. I'm trying not to be jealous, like I shouldn't be. She's leaning over to be cuddly with another guy, and she's leaning back to be caught. Am I the kind of guy that would feel that way? Now I'm with my brother. I go to climb in bed and my mother's soiled diaper and bugs are there. My brother says there are only gnats and you can't sleep against plastic. I finish that conversation and I say is there something you want? I say this to mother. And she takes it very badly. I try to get her to want something.*

My interpretation centered around his producing his own feelings, that is generating jealousy within himself to create distance rather than have contact with me and specifically depending upon the analytic work. He further produces a chain of causality by manufacturing feelings which have a palpable effect. He agreed to this and stated that that is what he means by "working things out for himself" and "getting my way." In terms of the issue of causality, I further detailed that the connection between his means of being able to establish a visual image or other sensory phantasy would produce a feeling as though his phantasy could lead to feeling in a direct causal form This process then produces an eventual sequence of phantasies and feelings. He could then feel that the contiguity of these mental events had a direct causal relation, one to the other, which then led to a quality of so-called "understanding," that further kept him in a capsular system in which he made the rules. The capsular system is represented by the cockpit in which he can no longer be perfectly enclosed in without severe "engineering difficulties." I continued, "Not only does he make the rules in this particular system, but that the words and the language that is utilized to speak to the outside world, in this instance myself, 'seems' to be articulate speech but in fact is an imitation of it organized for the purpose of generating a particular set of phantasies and feelings but also meant to keep a barrier between himself and myself."

A dream several weeks later further reveals a further stage of the presentation of imitative speech in a much less concrete way as many of the issues had achieved symbolic representation through the analytic work.

> A. *A youth is lean and bare-chested, worried about getting sun burned. I tell him we do not have to stay long after the sun comes up, one does not have to stay that long, and we'll do our work while we're there.*

B. *There is a three foot wall in the shape of an L. On either side of the wall, there is a game between single guys and single girls. A game show host is calling out the name Allan, and lots of guys respond to the name. Is it "cool" to lie? There can't be all that many Allans. I'm nervous about getting ready for when I get called on. I'm exposed and want to put on some underpants, so I see boxer shorts that have a hole in them, and I put them on over my shorts. They look okay. The guy that was being called on is asked his age. I don't want to tell. I would try to avoid making it an issue. I couldn't be natural about it.*

C. *The host starts to demonstrate what the guy had been called on to do. He is acting some part. Instantly, he's got tears. Then he's able to put on a laugh—I'm really surprised he's doing it. He's getting a lot of practice acting and I'm impressed. I say I'd hire him as an actor. There is a guy in front of me who is related to the host. I ask if it's his brother? He says it's his father. These guys look ethnic (Middle Eastern). He knows Yiddish and all sorts of Jewish stuff but he's not Jewish. He's learned all that stuff.*

D. *My friend B asks him what time Kaddish is? We'll do our version of it at the beach. This guy is dressed bizarrely, (the host). Layers of leotards, too small, not pulled up all the way like he's a fool. My mother would get stuck with her pants pulled down. Not on all the way.*

E. *Next I'm walking with my girlfriend who is very young and pretty and it's nice. We're young. There is a crowd of others and it's new. But I see "R," an old friend from high school. She is an experimental psychologist at Yale now and just got separated from Allan (in actuality). Suddenly I'd forgotten my girlfriend's name—I turn away to stall for time. I ask him questions about what her name is. I don't like that name. It begins with an "M". Melissa . . . Margaret . . . I go through the alphabet to see if that triggers something. A saleslady overhears the noises I am making and she thinks that there is something wrong. I say I'm just putting vowels and consonants together, trying to remember something. Trying to come up with the girl's name. (Here in my own countertransference experience I think remember-dismember.)*

F. *I massage the saleslady's back—she shows me some jewelry and tries to explain to me that my mom is making it hard for herself . . . to make selections about which jewels. My mother thinks she needs to look up the individual components . . . all the beads in the catalog in order to make a selection. If she were the manufacturer, that's what she'd have to do. Mom shows up with this piece looking like curly lettuce or a sea plant which is white . . . what they had on display wasn't white, it was clear transparent, so she found what she liked . . . . I admire that and it seems like a waste but if she doesn't buy things often, she's entitled to it. I'd come up with the idea to ask the store to hold it. Maybe it will talk her out of it but maybe it won't be lost. It cost a thousand dollars, but if it's given to my sister, she'll lose it in her junk or break it. She couldn't tell the difference between junk and valuable stuff and I can't tell the difference either.*

I am reporting a paraphrasing of interpretations of the dream interspersed with the dream text.

a. The confusion about work is represented. He feels he is being exposed to radiation which he is afraid will burn him (the analysis). He is told that the time, is short (that is life) and his exposure is limited, that is he can control the exposure, and that time is emerging as having meaning. The time of his life, suddenly relates to the time in a session. The limits of time being short as a model for the changing experience of life from infinite time to limited and particular time.

b. In the B section, there is a reference to the use of language in meeting women. (There has always been a terror of this and an "act" has been maintained.) Should he lie? He always has, and now it's just coming through to him, as he has always dated women 20 years or so younger and has been frustrated. He has been confused about this since he "looks" much younger and has been able to "act" in a such a way so that younger women think he is "cool," and timely (current style) to them (precisely how his father behaves at the age of 86) but he is afraid that the analytic process is catching him with his pants down so that he feels humiliated as a result of the discovery of his ruse to himself or the lie which produces embarrassment (bare ass) upon discovery. Boxer shorts are a reference to his martial arts stance in the transference and in life and feeling of a general fear that he will be discovered as a phony or an imitation.

c. The analytic process reveals to him his increasing awareness of his fabrication of reality to someone else (being someone or acting like someone he is not), an actor, and his continued confusion about his skill and use of acting. He gets lost in time while his friend, B, asks him what time Kaddish is, which is an appropriate use of a ritual but nonetheless an effective reference to death (an end to fabrication and a clear reference to facts). There are clear references to, his mother caught with her pants down, soiling, which she actually does, and the host father who acts big and dresses bizarrely—a fool—who also denies who he is and his age.

d. The wish to be young and happy with a nice, normal girlfriend is intruded upon by time again. The woman R, who represents a friend of 30 years ago in high school in actuality, is seen and shows up—suddenly he changes state of mind and gets confused. He forgets the young girl's name and tries to fabricate it out of sounds, vowels and consonants, going through the alphabet to see if it triggers something. He recognizes that for him speech is making infantile sounds without meaning. The saleslady, discovering something wrong, represents the part of him referencing communication to the outside as disordered and an imitation of human speech. "I'm just going through the vowels and consonants to remember the girl's name." These references clearly demonstrate an increasing awareness by the more developed part of himself identified with the analyst of problems that have reached enough significance to himself to be symbolized and apperceived.

e. Mother thinking that she needs to "look up all the original components, all the beads in the catalogue" illustrates a difficulty in trusting words as though one could better understand if all the letters or individual components could be compared in the "catalog-alphabet" in order to get them across as meaning (make or sell them). Language has been so defaced that there is the sense that it has to be invented anew. What can be added as creativity is doubted, as "creativity" cannot be distinguished from meaningless distortion.

f. There is an aspect of him identified with his mother who puts ideas together in an interesting way but is unable to use them as currency because their representation, although creative, is idiosyncratic and not suitable for use in communication as words are which accurately stand for something. Until now, these creations have been lost, but now they are close enough to be recognized as jewels which may

> have a use, not merely for decoration. They are valuable. Much of the communication actually spoken to his sister is misused or treated as junk and cannot be developed. If he could better differentiate between value and mental detritus, he could decide what to use and what is not valuable for communication. These are references to the products of his mind which represent the alpha elements suitable for use in symbol formation which can lead to unique jewels demonstrating his creativity if they were not mixed with other defaced and blunted aspects of mental process which make them indistinguishable from rubbish. He hopes that there can be a containment long enough to differentiate them through the analytic process and that he can store them so that they can be retrieved and differentiated. The sea plant looking like curly lettuce is not the same as that which they have on display (common use) for that is a reference to invention and it is also reference to the opacity of his use of language; that is, it is not clear like the one on display.

The problems with which the patient must deal involve fundamental difficulties in the formal operations of thinking. He must avoid contact to remain "encapsulated" yet the lysis of the barrier reveals to him increasing difficulties about verbal thought and communication. He faces the severe humiliation that he has "imitated human speech" making noises which, rather than communicating a precise symbolic meaning to himself and then to someone else, various substitutes occur. He has used verbal thought to induce visual phantasies which give him the image he wishes to believe and has remained deluded even throughout the analytic process which has demonstrated these delusions and hallucinations to him. He has realized that he believed he had to maintain these images to allay fears of catastrophic change and intensely painful affect which he could not tolerate. His use of "reversible perspective" (Bion, 1962) having been discovered by both of us hindered his use of it, yet evasion had to be maintained in order to avert catastrophe. Increasing awareness of his associations being evasions and lies led to intense pain, yet could only be given up in slow increments as his pain tolerance increased. The recognition of his use of imitative noises sounding like human speech has been grievously upsetting. His subsequent inability to value the analyst's communications because they utilize articulate speech which has never been trusted is a consequence. Vowels and consonants produce sounds which have an action, trigger memories, induce affects and images but have not been organized to stand for something and could not be confidently used to represent meaning.

This has led the patient to despair relating to his use of both conscious and unconscious insincerity. Severe difficulties with memory and the maintenance of continuity of thought are evident. These problems directly relate to the inability to "store" received verbal communication complicated by deflection of attention and degraded alpha elements only suitable for evacuation.

References to having to derive meaning from letters and the basic syllables of words are referred to in the dream material (mother thinking she needs to look up the individual components—all the beads in the catalogue to make a selection as though she were the manufacturer). Going through the alphabet to see if it triggers something demonstrates the kind of maneuver one sees in a Korsakoff's psychosis in which fabrications are utilized craftily to hide the fact that there is a gap in memory or blank in consciousness. The saleslady, overhearing his "noises," is an indicator that he is increasingly aware of his "putting vowels and consonants together" in a different way (again an imitation of speech). The saleslady represents an aspect of his personality organized to sell his language-act to the outer world, and when she acknowledges the apperceived difficulty, he massages her to seduce her (message/ massage), a primitive pun.

The references to the ethnic types who learned "all that Jewish stuff" involves contempt for those who mouth phrases and sounds in a language for which they have no understanding of the symbolic verbal content but pass off their use of sounds as though it were understanding. One can see the split attitude toward lying and the conscious "con job," that is the confidence game attitude which is felt to be far superior to the truth.

References to bringing together defaced elements of mother and father in verbal form involve a destructive, hateful version of the primal scene contributing to both the concretism and disordered creativity which plays a role in his mistrust of language.

Theoretical Links

I want to paraphrase and quote from W.R. Bion's (1955) "Language and the Schizophrenic." Bion referred to Freud's 1924 paper on "Neurosis and Psychosis" in which an, important distinction between these categories is made. "Neurosis is the result of a conflict between the ego and its id, whereas psychosis is the analogous outcome of a similar disturbance in the relation to the ego and its environment (outer world)" (p. 220). Bion reminds us that Freud's formula points to the psychotic patient's hostility to reality, and conflict with it, which enables us to grasp one element that determines the nature of endopsychic conflict.

In reference to Freud's 1911 article, "Formulations Regarding the Two Principles of Mental Functioning," Bion quotes,

> The increasing significance of external reality heightened the significance also of the sense organs directed toward that outer world, and of the consciousness attached to them; the latter now learned to comprehend the qualities of sense in addition to the qualities of pleasure and 'pain' which hitherto had alone been of interest to it (p. 221).

Bion states,

> It will be one of my contentions that the conflict with reality leads the psychotic patient to developments which make it doubtful whether he has ever learned to "comprehend the qualities of sense in addition to the qualities of pleasure and pain." Further, I shall suggest there is evidence which may indicate that destructive attacks have been directed by the patient, or the patient's id, against the newly significant sense organs and "the consciousness attached to them" (p. 221).

Bion continues:

> In my view, what Freud describes as the institution of the reality principle is an event that has never been satisfactorily achieved by the psychotic, and the main failure takes place at the point which Melanie Klein describes as the development of the depressive position. The reality principle, if it were allowed to operate, would make the psychotic infant aware of his relationship with whole objects, and thereby of the feelings of depression and guilt associated with the depressive position. It is at this point, however, that the patient makes destructive attacks on those aspects of his personality, his ego, that are concerned with establishing external contact and internal contact. What are these special aspects of the ego? Freud cites 1) attention; 2) notation, which he says is a part of that which we call memory; 3) an impartial passing of judgment; 4) a new function entrusted to motor discharge which is now concerned with action; and 5) restraint of action "by means of a process of thought which was developed from ideation" (p. 221).

Freud states:

> Thought was endowed with qualities which made it possible for the mental apparatus to support increased tension during a delay in the process of discharge. It is essentially an experimental way of acting, accompanied by displacement of smaller quantities, of cathexis together with less expenditure (discharge of them)" (p. 222).

Bion states that he thinks that all these special adaptations (except 4) are really aspects of the establishment of verbal thought; further, that this development is one aspect of the synthesizing and integrating forces which Melanie Klein has described as characteristic of the depressive position. Bion (1955) regards "disturbance in the development of verbal thought as an important aspect of psychosis, particularly, but not exclusively of schizophrenia" (p. 222). He continues,

> Castration of the ego is identical with destructive attacks on 1) the consciousness attached to the sense organs; 2) attention—the function which Freud says is instituted to search the outer world; 3) the system of notation which he describes as part of memory; 4) the passing of judgment which was developed to take the place of repression; and finally 5) thought as a way of supporting the increased tension produced by the restraint on motor discharge. With regard to this last point, I would add that in my view, verbal thought is the essential feature of all five functions of the ego and that the destructive attacks on verbal thought or its rudiments is inevitably an attack on all (p. 222).

Bion makes clear that he believes that the same oral, urethral, anal, and muscular sadism that Melanie Klein (1930) describes as typical of the attacks on the mother's body is an action against the ego. The "castration" of the ego then is manifested in extremely sadistic attacks on all the aforementioned ego functions. Especially relevant is the capacity to support frustration of motor discharge which is dependent upon the development of verbal thought of which the above-enumerated functions are particular aspects. "The splitting of verbal thought is carried out cruelly, and the attempts at synthesis which are typical in psychotics, as in others, of the depressive position are frustrated because the splits are brought together cruelly" (p. 223). Bion brings to the paper a final point which is unfortunately often ignored, that the splitting mechanism is brought into action to minister to the patient's greed and is therefore not simply an unfortunate catastrophe of the kind that occurs when the patient's ego is split in pieces as an accompaniment of his determination to split his objects; "it is the outcome of a determination which can be expressed verbally as an intention to be as many people as possible so as to be in as many places as possible, so as to get as much as possible, for as long as possible—in fact timelessly" (p. 223).

What has this all to do with the imitation of human speech? In accurate verbal thought, words are utilized to refer to something which has a common currency, either something which is thought or which is perceived as part of the external world. Then, an imitation of human speech would sound "like" real speech that has certain essential differences. It could betray the attacks on the ego's capacity for attention, notation, judgment, restraint on motor action and thought, in a more subtle way than would be evident in schizophrenia but would be less violently noticeable. Life in the encapsulated state for these individuals would follow in a less obvious way Freud's formula for psychosis since insulation from the outside world is the goal organized by the primordial conscience.

In Chapter 5, I described the "danger" signals of "psychic movement" and demonstrated the derailing or deflecting attacks organized to put a stop to the awareness of change. The attacks on the perceptual organs which Bion (1955) described so profoundly aid in the maintenance of a phantasy of a timeless hermetic seal. In critical observation of patients in this state of mind, it is clear that there are severe distortions of judgment based on failure to accurately perceive and process incoming stimuli. Attention and notation are seriously compromised as well by the attacks on perception. While these points are quite clear in a severely compromised individual, detecting the "problem of imitation" becomes more difficult when the encapsulated state is not so obvious. In this less obvious state, the capacity for attention can be quite developed but for the purpose of maintaining a distance from true contact in which there is penetration of the mind coming from the other. That is, it must "seem" as though there is contact, especially verbally, and that there is an intellectual process in operation which "satisfies" the other member of the pair or group in conversation that there has been a receipt of the communication and a response which is apposite. "Success" of the mimetic communication can be judged by the perpetrator by the lack of penetration or confrontation coming from the other. It is clear when the responder in this case, the psychoanalyst, does not accept at face value the distancing, off-point communication, and draws attention to the problem at hand. This operation may produce penetration to the point at which it becomes noticeable to the analysand and immediately ushers in a disturbing resistance, either a full stop or a kind of defensive explosion organized to reestablish the hermetic seal by distancing the analyst and the language of true effect. This can appear as a form of the negative therapeutic reaction in which the patient will typically miss sessions or even bolt the analysis. As can be seen, this kind of confrontative analytic work takes considerable skill and that the progress jerks in starts and stops, the patient moving away from contact. Robert Caper (1995) has referred to noticing in the countertransference an anxiety as to whether one should make the interpretation which can be foreseen by the analyst to lead to a disturbance. It is as if the patient has said, "Here's the line and don't you dare cross it or else!" This hostility is definitely a function of the psychic pain and disorientation produced by the penetrating interpretation.

Bion (1955) makes the point clear that the development of verbal thought is a function of the integrative processes described by Melanie Klein (1930) as the depressive position. There is the immediate pain brought on by the awareness of guilt and lost time as well as the anxiety relating to needing an object that can abandon one, linked to the awareness of having damaged that object. In Bion's example (1955), the recognition of insanity is brought about by the analytic process and specifically by the development of verbal thought that is felt by the patient to have led to the difficulties. The depressive position emerges and the hatred of recognition of his delusions and hallucinated mental life occurs. The analyst must be prepared for severe emotional storms at this point and "concentrate on not allowing the patient to retreat from his realization that he is insane or from his hatred of the analyst who has succeeded, after so many years, in bringing him to an emotional realization of the facts which he has spent his life trying to evade" (p. 235).

Chapter 10

Transformational Aspects of Phantasy in Relation to Dyadic Communication under the Influence of Marijuana

Methods and General Problem

The purpose of this investigation is to develop a method for the study of altered states of consciousness in relation to internal phantasy and different forms of anxiety. The concept of altered states of consciousness will be enlarged to include altered psychosomatic considerations and to study aspects of the phenomena of communication as a consequence of marijuana administration. Although this study refers specifically to a state of consciousness induced by marijuana, it should be understood that the drug is being used as a tool for studying a series of altered states of consciousness as amplifications of basal states of mind. We will strive to describe changes of functioning in the psychological interpretation of data impinging upon the perceptual apparatus which correspond to the simultaneous state of drug intoxication induced by marijuana.

Cannabis sativa is widely known to produce an altered state of consciousness as are many other compounds with target effects in the central nervous system (Lemberger, Axelrod, and Kopin, 1972). Are the "mental effects" observable under such conditions simply the result of drug action causing biochemical and/or neurophysiological changes, or are they primarily the result of the immediate psychological effects related to set, philosophical frame of reference of subject, the psychological interpretation of primary autonomic phenomena induced by taking the drug, the social conditioning, the subject's state of consciousness, the fluctuations of extrinsic mood in the milieu, or as is highly likely, varying combinations of the above in addition to many other unmentioned variables?

We will attempt to describe the technique for the analysis of data received from videotape communication from a psychological point of view. The subjects are male, the time course of the period of intoxication under examination by videotape is constant, they receive a dose of marijuana and they talk. The setting is constant which consists of a simulated lounge with two television cameras fixed on the subjects who are seated in comfortable chairs but cannot see the cameras as they are hidden well. There is a monitor in the room which is visible as well as an overhanging microphone. This setting is conducive to a situation in which the subjects perceive themselves to be watched by an invisible eye, that they know is there. Thus we are observing a situation occurring between three basic points of reference, from the point of view of the camera as well as the two subjects. The state of being watched by an eye is a situation which occurs from birth onward, and there is always the presence of either an external object watching, or the phantasy of an internal object. We have observed generally that there is considerable use of the "us-them" concept which is useful to describe the variations in emotional linking, but is influenced by the setting. "Then I am an actor. But it's funny, it also feels like someone is still watching me. So it's really funny in a way, even though we are not supposed to, I feel like we're a team of actors doing something right over there . . . Us and them." (Laughter.) This is the first statement of one of the pair of intoxicated subjects after sitting in the studio a minute or so. In that we are dealing with a setting in an institution, we assume that some degree of suspicion exists because of the geometry of the room as well as being part of a government study. We thus record a ten minute segment initially in a nonintoxicated state so that we have a comparison to the altered state of consciousness produced by the drug.

Each subject receives a standard dosage of 7 mg THC (9 tetrahydrocannabinol—active principle of marijuana) per kilogram/body weight contained in government grown marijuana which has been assayed shortly before use to contain approximately 4% THC. Each cigarette contains approximately 400 to 500 mg of marijuana calculated according to body weight. The study was designed as a double blind and the groups which receive marijuana stripped of Δ-9-THC were decoded after statistical analysis.

We are studying syntactical patterns of verbal productions considered as phantasy. When we use the word phantasy we refer to a transformative process beginning with preverbal, inchoate, presymbolic experience involving sense data received from the outside and following this material through a continuum of increasing abstraction to a symbolic verbal production. In this context we wish to relate phantasy to an understanding of internal mental space in which the specific phantasy represents an attempt to cope with a conflict which reveals itself as a symbolic form of mental work. The function of this work is to comprehend (locate) symbolically the issues concerned and to transform them to a more utilizable form and location. To be experienced, the transformation can only be perceived when movement has occurred, gaining separation in mental space and perspective from another vertex. (This is a mental representation of coping with an issue.) In other words, experience is taken in, in one form, and transformed into another system of comprehension. Phantasy then becomes a means for understanding experience, which is a complex way of spatially locating sense data and making them available in a symbolic form. Phantasy may refer to a process occurring consciously or unconsciously. Narratives or stories used as material by the subjects then are considered to pertain to the situation occurring at the moment between the subjects. What is used as "real information" then, based on "fact" is defined as phantasy which we consider as data in this investigation. This technique is by no means new but is used in the psychoanalytic context to understand the relationship between analyst and analysand.

What is written here then, is a condensation of the thought process evoked in the minds of the observers which is mutually corroborated.

In this study we have the advantage of producing a change in the mental set of the subjects which is termed intoxication. Furthermore we can say that the process has to do with marijuana, the dosage of which can be correlated with considerable statistical significance to the subjective assessment of the degree of intoxication by the user. Since we study experienced smokers there exists a high degree of agreement between the subjects about their level of intoxication which they attribute to marijuana. Therefore, we are dealing with a substance known to the subjects, to produce a change in the state of consciousness which is endowed with certain views or phantasies. Further, it is taken into the body by deep inhalation and is, in fact, within the body producing a subjective effect changing over time for a period of hours. Indeed it is not completely excreted from the body for somewhat over nine days (Lemberger, Axelrod, and Kopin, 1972). Often in the context of this experience, strong feelings emerge either consciously or unconsciously which we observe to have profound effects upon the relationship of the subjects. Love, hatred, envy, and anxiety are included in the intense affects that must be considered. We deliberately raise these issues relating to the partition of intoxication between phantasy and drug effect, since any study of this nature which is by necessity nonquantitative and impossible to "control" within the context of ordinary scientific methodology, could be profitably be considered. It seems evident that there are myriad variant conditions by which any study involving human subjects are hindered. Thus we are noting what we consider to be constantly conjoined elements which seem to come together again and again in order to develop theory about the underlying phenomena producing these organized patterns.

Definitions of Gap and the Functions of Phantasy

We are studying a form of anxiety which presents itself whenever one becomes aware of separation between the self and another. We will refer to this experience of separation either consciously or unconsciously as the gap. The awareness of a gap results in a state of anxiety. The presence of a gap between two persons involved in this field of relationship is the paradigm in one direction, but in equilibrium with this state is a condition of actively attempting to obliterate this gap. The gap stimulates a form of anxiety which has to do with the awareness that another person has what is experienced as something that is needed. Thus the perception of need both stimulates the awareness of the gap and the simultaneous attempt to obliterate it. It is our impression from these experiments that this process occurs in phasic motion as if one were observing a hole to the void open, shut and partially open revealing dread in different dosages. It is our observation that this phantasied hole, as it were, is experienced as the stimulus for intense anxiety. Thus, there is negotiation of this hole by a single individual mediated by parts of the personality, solipsistically, and in concert with the interactional group which may be another personality and/or a series of other persons. If the latter point is considered, the situation occurring between two persons is phenomenologically complex. We then may consider the "field effect" of a "feeling" of psychological pain related to the perception of absence, although in most instances unrecognized, in the space between persons to be considered as an interactional matrix.

Envy-in-the-Field Associated with the Use of Marijuana

One may consider a set of phenomena occurring in the separate individuals as one compartment in the system, and a different set of phenomena occurring in the space between the group members taken as another unit in the system. We will use the word "envy" to describe a measure of the inability to tolerate the unwanted awareness of the absence of that which is experienced as needed. Initially there exists a state of anxiety which may result in the obliteration of the perception of need or the individual containing the object of need. This process of obliteration (spoiling) is referred to by Klein and her co-workers as an envious attack (Klein, 1957). Envy may be present in a varying dose, existing in the field between, changing with time, either in or out of awareness, palpable or not as a form of anxiety. In this study we will deal primarily with this unrecognized form of envy hitherto undistinguishable from anxiety. We have observed anxiety handled through action without thought often coupled with autonomic discharge through the peripheral sympathetic and parasympathetic nervous system in which the outflow state may be studied under the heading of stress. We posit the hypothesis that there exists in this context a separate and undischargeable form of anxiety which persists in the "field" which for the sake of convenience we name protoenvy and which represents that form of anxiety which cannot be released (evacuated) through action without thought.

To illustrate this situation we will consider a two person system in which intense anxiety associated with a drug effect, exists in the matrix of the field between the persons. This anxiety is not dealt with by locomotory flight because of the experimental set. Action by locomotion then is minimized, then speech may be used as a form of action in addition to its symbolic use. If we consider this action as an attempt by one group member at unburdening his psyche of this state of anxiety into the field of the other in order to annihilate the perception of the gap (hole), then group member B is to some extent the recipient of this anxiety in an unspoken way. We mean by this that neither A nor B has conscious awareness that the state of affairs stated above is occurring. It is, nevertheless, felt as a state of anxiety, described in drug user parlance as one form of "bad vibes."(A reference to the idea that one can experience "emanations" or a "vibrational energy" coming from the other. This vibration is subjectively felt to originate in the other and be sent across the gap as if it were a particle. It must be stated that while there is evidence of a kind for this experience, we cannot prove its existence with methodology developed as of this time.) There may be on B's part an attempt to contain this state or as frequently is observed, a need to eject this unwelcome experience. We are describing a process of communication in abstracted form which describes a set of frequently observed variations in perception by two group members. The currency for this interaction is verbal communication, thus agents of conveyance for these "bad vibes" are words strung together in narrative form although the communication elaborated by one member A, may be phantasy containing symbolic meaning, it also serves the function of filling the gap as a method of denying the perception of separation between A and B from A's point of view. If the purpose of this communication is to annihilate A's perception of the gap in reference to B, the form of action taken by this communication would involve blocking A's perception of B (or what had previously stated) which had induced a state of protoenvy in A. B's statement which evoked A's blocking narrative would then be met with a form of annihilation, stripping, or desymbolization and B might apprehend this by experiencing A as devaluing or spoiling his communication. If B is using his statement as a technique for projecting a part of his personality into the field, then B would experience this stripping process as an attack upon his person. This state of affairs may or may not be in B's awareness. Therefore, B's response may be immediate or delayed depending upon the number of corrosive attacks needed to produce awareness on some level of the nature of his experience. Thus in this situation B may attack A assuming that A is hostile. A, however, may not be aware of B's experience and is operating in a defensive maneuver elaborated to annihilate the gap. This represents one kind of dysjunctional experience in hypothetical terms to serve as a model for the use of a theoretical system.

In the dialogue of the experience stated above, we have made use of several concepts developed in other contexts such as (1) the use of verbal productions as a form of action (Freud, 1911; Bion, 1955, 1962), (2) the progressive concretization and stripping of the symbol (verbal communication in this context) (Bion, 1962; Klein, 1957), and (3) a form of the Kleinian theory of projective identification in an attempt to extend the concept of envy (Klein, 1957). By projective identification, we mean a phantasied extrusion of a partial self-representation and the consequent creation of mental space, with the experience of the loss of the self-representation and/or one's object representations along with this self-representation.

We have observed in a series of pairs of subjects under the influence of marijuana, phenomena we have introduced up to this point as amplification of the experience of the feelings which come up in communication between two persons. Among these feelings we have noted intense anxiety, hatred, contempt, a need to cling to the other, intimidation and reaching out to join. We feel that these phenomena represent the experience of a rapid amplification of the process occurring between two persons. As a result of this amplified experience in addition to other factors discussed below such as translocation of affect and/or parts of the personality in phantasy, defensive maneuvers are elaborated. We have noted a number of phenomena including contempt for the other, hatred, stripping the meaning from the statements of one of the members of the pair, bound in common by their effect of spoiling the communication of the other. These factors have been previously noted to be associated with envy. It is assumed then, that these factors are the results of envy-in-the-field between the subjects. As a result of this state of mental affairs, a defensive posture is seen to develop. Further, under these conditions there has been observed a progressive concretization of thought and hence verbal communication. Associated with these factors, envy and concretization of thought, we have noted severe anxiety as well as phantasied loss of distinction between group members.

Modes of Defense in Phantasy

We have previously described a state of mind in which the awareness of the gap leads to severe anxiety based upon the dread of possible extinction (awareness of helplessness and need for an object). This state of awareness of helplessness and need has been associated with the beginnings of orality (Freud, 1905). The aspects of need, dependency and the anxiety of separation exist from the point of the initial contact with the other individual and can be described in oral, anal, and genital modes (Erikson, 1964). Phantasy is used in this form of experience to change zonal modes from one in which the awareness of the separation (gap) between the group members leads to severe anxiety based on the awareness of helplessness and need, and which may be called a form of orality to a defensive posture against this impotent state by changing the mode to an anal zone (location) in which there is the perception by the subject of at least some form of control.

To illustrate this process we have selected a segment from a session between subjects X and Y in which there is concern suddenly for their use of language. The question arises how we, the observers, must be considering their very frequent use of certain words, e.g., "shit." "X" states, "Well, they'll conclude from this that dopers say shit and fuck a lot. They are listening to our mind process." "X" states, "I was digging around in the back room amidst all the machines and it freaked me out." At this time the subjects are smoking and report at least partial intoxication. This phantasy was taken as demonstrative of an anal mode in which invasion was occurring on the part of "X." This subject has located himself in phantasy in the lower end of the gastrointestinal tract corresponding to the anus or rectum (back room) and is experiencing persecutory anxiety ("It freaked me out") in relation to his invasion ("I was digging around").

It is our experience, utilizing this representative of many phantasies associated with marijuana use in this study, that a form of anatomical zonal confusion (Meltzer, 1966) results. The equation of self with the mother (in infantile terms) as a ploy to deny separation is noted here. This represents, in our experience, a defense against separateness, feelings of envy, helplessness, and exposure to being seen as vulnerable. Thus the phantasy has transformed an oral situation into a defense against perception of need by utilizing an anal mode. To avoid the helplessness brought about by the perception of the gap, there is confusion between the breast (of the mother), anus and mouth resulting in the interchangeability of food and feces. The buttocks and feces (the products thereof) become confused with the breast and the milk. In this unit of phantasy in the experimental situation, it is felt that they have taken inside an internal observer, i.e. primitive form of mother, who can see more than they. They have introjected the camera as a representation of an all-seeing internal object in the form of the experimentalist-mothers who are felt to be viewing it, as if we are experienced as knowing all that they know and more. To lose one's private boundary in this context is to be "freaked out." To state the situation differently: there is no space between them and us because the eye (camera) has penetrated the subject from his point of view. In their view, they are taking "shit" inside them and are seen by the observers with their shit. Thus to be known is to be in contact with bad shit. This may represent a prototype of a psychosomatic defensive function noted in phantasy. The marijuana is equated by the subjects with the good feeding situation but is "stolen" in phantasy such that it is necessary to disguise the valuable food by calling it shit, so they won't be discovered. Thus the phantasy has transformed an oral situation into a defense against this perception of need by utilizing an anal mode. We are here observing an anal defensive system of phantasy. What controls this system which is being invoked and what are the determining factors in inducing the shift from one zonal mode to another?

The next point in this videotape referred to a phantasy of drug effectiveness. A states, "The more of them I smoke, the stonder I get!" B states, "On this? Oh, yeah! It's not like parsley or something." B continues, "Like if you would smoke parsley for twenty years, you probably wouldn't get high any more. Know what I mean? Like, if now we could smoke one and get a little high, but in ten or twenty years, we'd have to smoke twenty of them to get a little high." A states, "O.K., it doesn't work that way. I don't think. I know the first time you smoke it, it takes a hell of a lot. The more you smoke, the less it takes, but at first, you probably reach a point of vanishing returns and you just can't smoke any less."

Identification of Feeling State Which is Known to Cohere Phantasy

This segment of phantasy represents a view of the gap between the two. In this phantasy segment there are elements suggesting a search for a concrete representation of the symbol for the original experience of contact which is achieved somatically with the drug. There is acknowledgment of a state of familiarity with the "feeling" of intoxication (referred to as "high") that is learned as a physical sensation with the suggestion that with increasing experience less and less of the drug is necessary to accomplish the task of achieving this "feeling." There is prevailing anxiety that motivates the subjects to locate the "danger" through a sensuous experience in that the anxiety is not discernible in a sensuous form, e.g. as a physical sensation like being touched. There is a need to convert an intuitive experience (a feeling of anxiety) into a somatic experience. The subjects cannot locate their dread produced as a result of their relation to the gap. They sense the experience of separation but cannot comprehend it therefore there is a conversion into a somatic sensation. Thus, it is put into the more primary "language" of somatic sensations. The "feeling" the subjects are in contact with is an effect felt to be "knowable" to them. Here they have mastered their experience of separation by the phantasied contact, induced by the perception of the drug effect, with that which is not comprehended. The gap (experience of separation) creates for them an impasse in locating the necessary object. They have made nothing into something in phantasy through the drug experience. This maneuver may be an attempt to reverse the forces of envy. They are trying to convert an absence experience, a result of the gap, to a concrete "physical" experience.

Premature loss is experienced as a catastrophe. There is a search for a sensuous feeling to put them in phantasied contact with the needed thing. After contact with the drug effect is achieved, the subject can "recognize" and master that which is experienced as lost by evacuative control. In this manner, they can then "create" the gap under their control. There is a controlled separation; "I'm not fired, I quit." These maneuvers are representative of an anal mode which is the defense against an "oral" anxiety situation, that of loss of a needed object. The thought is dismantled and the "feeling" remains as a return to primary process.

This is a method of warding off the experience of the separation leading to protoenvy. Two different techniques by which anality is achieved are observed; one by mastery and control of the phantasied absent object and the other by desymbolization of the meaning of need. The corrosive effect of protoenvy induces anality by desymbolizing (concretizing) the meaning of need and/or the source of the food, be it milk, or its counterpart-food for thought. The dismantling of the symbol results in the mental equivalent of feces which is a specific phantasied psychosomatic defense against the perception of need. This process alters the meaning of the symbol such that it can be used for other mediums of exchange. We suggest here that our subjects are defending against their own emptiness by murdering the perception of the gap, which is the result of protoenvy. This form of envy may be a biological inborn awareness *of* one's own limitations. Is envy an attempt to obviate internalized extinction anxiety? If so, this form of anxiety is premised upon the awareness that one cannot adequately meet the needs of the self without the presence of a feeding object. This serves as a form of antiomnipotent interpretation coming from the outside. If envy is to be defended against by a form of phantasy, it becomes clear that the elaboration of phantasy assumes an anal mode to develop a *form* of "food" suitable to simulate the outside, e.g., by the sensuous experience of the drug. Thus, filling the hole with phantasied feces represents an attempt at bypass of the awareness of the gap utilizing the verbal productions as a plastic medium either to use as currency to buy off the perception of the hole or to degrade the other person, in the interaction. To be without the symbol in this context is to be in contact with the void (viewed as death), or as in our example above is equivalent to "being freaked out." The psychotic in the state of concretization of thought cannot symbolize. Therefore, he is aware of vast spaces or holes, putting him more in contact with massive envy which is defended against by the annihilation of the gap.

We are describing two methods of dealing with the gap (see *Figure 10.1.*) One is constructive, leading to symbolization, learning from experience and growth while the second method leads to concretization, desymbolization and evacuation of symbolic content and meaning.

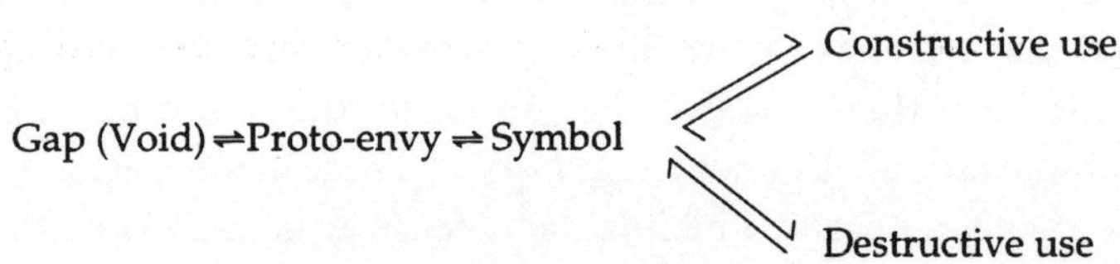

Figure 10.1

Defenses Function Against Protoenvy

We have discussed in terms of protoenvy a beginning state of distinguishing between primitive forms of anxiety and the attempt to discover qualitative differences in form which relate to function. To locate "content" in terms of the use of the symbol may be a function of protoenvy which puts the subject in contact with an experience of the void or gap.

When these functions are viewed in terms of mental equilibria, the gap may be perceived as the substrate for the development of the symbol. Inherent in any symbol is the process of delimiting an experience in the form of a sense impression originally kept out of awareness in undigested and unusable form. These experiences can become usable when they are transformed into thought. Bion, in *Learning from Experience*, makes the point that such "experiences" (beta elements) are "not amenable to use in dream thoughts but are suited for use in projective identification" (p. 6). He continues, "They are objects that can be evacuated or used for a kind of thinking that depends on manipulations of what are felt to be things-in-themselves as if to substitute such manipulation for words or ideas" (p. 6). In other words, this form of thinking represents action without thought, *not a contemplative process.*

The differential between the symbol and thing-in-itself (that which can only be known by its primary and secondary qualities) is the distance or space from the concrete to the representation of the concrete.

Hanna Segal (1956) in "Notes on symbol formation" states,

> Symbol formation is an activity of the ego attempting to deal with the anxieties stirred up by its relation to the object. That is primarily the fear of bad objects and the fear of the loss or inaccessibility to good objects (p. 392).

She continues,

> In particular, disturbances in differentiation between ego and object lead to disturbances in differentiation between the symbol and the object symbolized and therefore to concrete thinking characteristic of psychosis (p. 393).

Further,

> In the symbolic equation the symbol substitute is felt to *be* the original object. The substitute's own properties are not recognized or admitted. The

> symbolic equation is used to deny the absence of the ideal object, or to control a persecuting one (*ibid.*).
>
> But,
>
> . . . the symbol proper available for sublimation and furthering the development of the ego, is felt to represent the object; its own characteristics are recognized, respected and used . . . (*ibid.*).
>
> The symbol is used not to deny but to overcome loss. When the mechanism of projective identification is used as a defense against depressive anxieties, symbols already formed and functioning as symbols may revert to symbolic equations (*ibid.*).

We refer to the form of anxiety designated by the term protoenvy as existing either as the result of degradation of the symbol to a thing-in-itself or before the symbolic equation is apprehended for use in negotiating the gap between the self and the object. Thus it is at the interface, between the gap and its negotiation, that the symbolic equation is generated. We hypothesize that to be without at least a symbolic equation, in lieu of a symbol, dread or the experience of not being exists. To the infant, this experience of the gap without symbol is provocative of extinction anxiety (later developed as the fear of death).

In lieu of a symbol we have seen return to the bodily sensation via the drug which may be the interface phenomenon representing the beginning of a psychosomatic experience.

If one loses contact with the awareness of the sensory apparatus and is put in contact with simulated endless space, a form of severe anxiety is present. Experiments producing sensory deprivation have demonstrated the development of a psychotic state and may shed light on the problem of symbol formation. Sense impressions may be thought to be precursors to the symbol, some form of memory representation employing a perceptual sense. Without the symbol, there lacks a form of boundary which structures or locates the limits of space. The symbol is used mentally as a representation of something physical, a link bringing together something which has a sensory actuality to something, which has not, like a thought or an idea. Verbal thought may then be dependent upon symbol formation. As the ability to utilize verbal thought diminishes or is retarded, so is the ability to negotiate the gap which involves the development of anxiety. If there is fluctuation in the relative use of verbal thought induced, perhaps, by a drug such as marijuana, then there is repeated exposure to the gap occurring with a periodicity. The question whether or not this anxiety (gap) summates is of importance qualitatively. If the anxiety reaches and exceeds a threshold, projective identification (phantasied fusion and invasion) may occur to reduce this gap. Projective identification results in entrapment in the extreme leading to the development of severe anxiety and withdrawal based on a persecutory experience. Thus one may see oscillation between one form of anxiety due to phantasied invasion, and a form of anxiety based on the persecution form of anxiety related to the lack of use of the symbol secondary to anxiety in the context of protoenvy. This oscillation may be what is referred to as the "bum trip."

Bion (1967) has related a theory of thinking based on the model of the alimentary canal. In this context symbols may have an "anal origin." By this we mean that the first awareness of internal space has to do with eating, voiding and defecation. The creation of internal space by the infant may be the result of defecation which on a process involving loss of a concrete thing. This involves a change in the frame of reference of space (the gap) from the inside to the outside in terms of a representation of the psychic view of the internal. The term "anal" in this context refers to that change in frame of reference from the mouth to the anus and out. This is a process which definitely evolves in time. Thus inherent in any symbol is the representation of time. The symbol may be described, then, as locating time which delimits anxiety. The symbol represents a primitive form of reassurance in helping the individual to locate himself (to find a boundary) in a timeless dimension.

Protoenvy Can Lead to Definition of a Symbol

Protoenvy locates *the* symbol in the *other* of what is wanted for the self. The symbol is partially the result of this protoenvy in that what is perceived in the other is possessed by the self in the form of the symbol representing what is absent or lacking. One may avoid the perception of time and space by appropriating the function of the symbol, indeed partially fusing with it. Proportional to the degree of fusion of the self representation with the symbol, action develops out of thought. The greater the degree of this fusion, the more action ("acting out") occurs without thought. Symbolic realization leads to action enabling the individual to cope with the anxiety related to protoenvy. If thinking in the extreme, is opposed to action, thinking presents the maximum use of the symbol with the greatest distance from it. Perhaps thought does not involve the process understood by what we call verbal thinking. Here one may be dealing with what Jung termed an archetype or a preconception which once mated with a sense impression becomes a symbol.

PROTO-ENVY

Symbolization	**Locomotion without symbolization**
Gap awareness	**Dimished gap awareness**
Action with thought	**Action without thought**
Location of the mind in space	**Dread and location of the body in space**
(Triangulation through phantasy)	**Relative internal spacelessness**
Development and growth based on mobility of symbolic recombination	**Relocation of thought in the form of action (memory in physiological terms)**

LOCATION

Figure 10.2

This schema (*Figure 10.2*), although crude, represents a beginning attempt to understand the "psychosomatic" aspects of the anlage of proto-envy as we have described the process thus far. In drug user parlance, one hears of the marijuana experience being described as either "body trip" primarily or a "head trip." By this, it is generally meant that the subject has an awareness of a process occurring on a somatic level, or a predominant experience of an intellectual journey, taking the form of phantasy. The awareness of this gap, stimulated by protoenvy, leads to different techniques for localization of the self in a "space-time-unit." Here, psyche and soma are used in conjunction in the differentiation of self from object.

> Confidence is a concomitant of knowing that there is full relation between the senses, or that more than one person in a group entertains what appears to be the same statement of the same representation of an emotional experience (Bion, 1962, p. 50).

Bion continues,

> Confidence in a representation is associated with 1) a belief that the representation is supported by common sense, and 2) that it not only represents the emotional experience from which it is abstracted, but represents other realizations, unknown when the abstraction was accomplished (*ibid.*).

Further,

> abstraction, then, can be seen as a step in publication which facilitates correlation by comparison of the representation. It has been abstracted with a number of different realizations, none of which is the realization in which the representation was originally abstracted. The concretization, by contrast, can be seen as a form of publication which facilitates correlation by common sense; that is, stating something so that it is recognized as an object of one sense, that can be tested as an object of another sense (*ibid.*).

Here, Bion has elaborated a theory for localizing an object in space by the application and integration of different sense data. Must we have psychic and somatic localization combined to have the perception of "control"? This control is represented by the presence of rheostatic adjustment of perception coming from somatic sources, which may or may not be in awareness, and the impression coming from "psychic sources" similarly is *in* or out of awareness. At what point are linkages established between psyche and soma? Following our previous schema, protoenvy must have a positive function in stimulating the awareness of the gap, in that it facilitates that formation and/or use of the symbol. It is as if there are either two forms of protoenvy or at least two described functions for the process. We must be then interested in the process in which this form of anxiety is used in relation to the symbol for constructive or destructive purposes, as mentioned above. The processing of anxiety which relates to Bion's formulation of a beta element involves the transformation of a previously unsymbolized proto thought into usable thought units or alpha elements. This process may have somatic connection in that not knowing where a body part is localized in space without thought may stimulate thought in order to obviate this situation. Entrapment may facilitate this transformation of beta into alpha function or proto thought to thought in that there is in the moment of entrapment, suddenly a limit around the nondelimited, infinite, dimensionless condition. The relationship to an object may provide containment. Thus, in this context, one cannot have "thoughts" without the anxiety we have designated, protoenvy. Here, the question, "can one have thought in a boundaryless environment?" becomes important. If one is deprived of a situation which creates a boundary, there is no perception of self, and this leads to massive anxiety. This massive anxiety may be what has been called "dread" in other contexts involving the loss of a boundary as a form of sensory deprivation, with the mobilization of a primitive form of envy, which opens the door, as it were, to the void (gap). In the moment that protoenvy allows "perception" of the gap (infinite space), there is potentiation of the already dimensionless situation present to some degree induced by the loss of perception stimulated by projective identification. Both systems combined, the loss of a boundary and the experience of protoenvy, lead to dread. Are the defenses against dread the same as against protoenvy? One form of anxiety seems to lead to autonomic discharge, a locomotor response, evacuation somewhat related to projective identification, whereas the second form of protoenvy leads to the experience of entrapment, in turn, leading to symbol formation, which then has variability, depending upon the use of the symbol. In the first system, the body or a body part is the symbol in which the individual is massively identified with his own "beta function," in which thoughts and things are felt to be interchangeable. One cannot separate the thought from the sensory experience in this context. The *body is the symbolic* equation in this context. The second system is contemplative, in that one is contained, and there is a need to use the symbol in order to get out of the container in phantasy. Protoenvy stimulates the development of the second system, which may include attack, which is usually called envy in the Kleinian frame of reference, and search (in phantasy) which is used to describe mental space. The propelling force in either method has at its base the purpose of locating the self. The question arises here, "what is necessary for the comprehension of mental space with boundaries?" We can study this by observing the process of the loss of the boundary. A description of a process of perception involves the discovery of different locations (spaces), so that one does not perceive the gap until there has been the perception of the loss or partial loss of what filled it. One locates a space not by the process of "having" it, but rather by the awareness of the presence of the absence of what filled the location before the loss. The concept of dimension, as in sculpture, has to do with understanding the form through loss or removal. Loss always seems to involve the development of protoenvy. Perception becomes the common denominator for the understanding of dimension. That which is perceived is retained in a distinctive form for each individual, but is not located or utilizable for thought until it is mated with a sense impression which implies something not self. The nearer one gets to a concretization of the symbol, the less there is a sense of dimensionality. The experience of receptivity to impinging sense data is dependent upon the existence of an external physical gap which then yields the mental representation of that which is not self. The very existence of even the beginning of the perception of a gap leads to protoenvy. The symbol provides the means to maintain the mental representation of the gap simultaneous with the ability to negotiate it in relation to either an internal or external object. The toleration of the gap is dependent upon the capacity to substitute the lost object and its contents with internal representations. The absence of symbolic capacity, then, is related to boundless space. If loss is equivalent mentally to death, then the death experience (gap) is warded off by discovering a substitute for what has been lost, which is the symbolic representation. The gap is necessary in order to develop the symbol. The symbol contains the representation of the gap and the invariant of the lost object (that which is outside the self) which created the gap. Thus, the symbol bridges the gap by substitution with an invariant process. Thought which is dependent upon the use of symbols requires the invariant process which allows for progression to increasing levels of abstraction.

In this chapter we have introduced an application of the psychoanalytic method applied to dyads by which an attempt has been made to elucidate a theory of the interaction of phantasy, utilizing marijuana as an amplifier of mental processes. By utilizing a psychoanalytic frame of reference, we have observed the development of the mental representation of the gap (states of separation leading to self-definition), and the attempt to negotiate or obliterate it through the mechanism of what we have termed protoenvy. The gap is experienced in one form, and transformed into another system of comprehension through the symbol. Phantasy becomes a means for understanding experience involving spatial location of sense data making them available for thought. As a consequence, we were able to study anxiety that came up as a consequence of the perception of separation between members of the pair. As a result, we were able to observe the "field effect" of a feeling of psychological pain resulting from the perception of absence and to conceptualize envy as a measure of the inability to tolerate the unwanted experience of the absence of what is experienced as needed. We have observed a shift in zonal modes, from "oral to anal," as a symbolic expression operating as a defense against the perception of the gap. We have noted the repeated search for a sensous experience via the use of marijuana, to reactivate the possibilities for discovering new symbols to reduce the anxiety of the gap. The marijuana experience may illustrate the prototype of a psychosomatic phenomenon the purpose for which may be to defend against the anxiety generated by the gap by returning to the sensuous experience prior to separation. This is an attempt to deny the gap by holding on to the sensory experience. In lieu of the symbol, the sensory experience is adhered to. In this context we have noted a fusion between the symbol and the object symbolized resulting in a high degree of concrete thinking. This has important implications for learning from experience, as well as for communication.

References

Argyle, M. (1972). Non-verbal communication in human social interaction. In Hinde, R.A. (Ed.), *Non Verbal Communication.* Cambridge and New York: Cambridge University Press, 243-.

Bion, W.R. (1955). Language and the schizophrenic. In *New Directions in Psycho-Analysis.* London: Tavistock Pubns., 220-239.

—— (1959). Attacks on linking. In *Second Thoughts.* London: Heinemann, 93-109.

—— (1962). *Learning from Experience.* London: Heinemann.

—— (1963). *Elements of Psycho-Analysis.* London: Heinemann.

—— (1965). *Transformations.* New York: Basic Books.

—— (1967). *Second Thoughts.* London: Heinemann.

—— (1970). *Attention and Interpretation.* London: Tavistock Pubns.

—— (1973). Personal conversations.

—— (1975). Lecture, Los Angeles Psychoanalytic Society, June 4, 1975.

—— (1977). Two Papers: *The Grid* and *Caesura.* Salomao, J. (Ed.). Rio de Janeiro: Imago Editora Ltd., pp. 43-58.

—— (1980). *Bion in New York and Sao Paulo.* Bion, F. (Ed.). Perthshire, Scotland: Clunie Press.

Brazelton, T.B., Koslowski, B., and Main, M. (1973). Early mother-infant reciprocity. In Lewis, M., Rosenblum, L. (Eds.), *The Origins of Behavior.* New York: Wiley, pp. 49-76.

—— (1975). Early mother-infant reciprocity. *CIBA Foundation Symposium* 33: *Parent-Infant Interaction.* New York: Associated Scientific Publishers.

Caper, R. (1995). On the difficulty of making a mutative interpretation. *Int. J. Psycho-Anal.*, 76: 91-101.

Chomsky, N. (1957). *Syntactic Structures.* The Hague: Mouton.

—— (1968). *Language and Mind.* New York: Harcourt, Brace and World.

Condon, W.S. and Sander, L.W. (1974). Neonate movement is synchronized with adult speech: interactional participation and language acquisition. *Science*, 183: 99-101.

Eisenberg, R.B. (1976). *Auditory Competence in Early Life.* Baltimore: University Park Press.

Erikson, E. (1964). *Childhood and Society.* 2nd Ed. New York: Norton.

Freud, S. (1900). *The Interpretation of Dreams. SE*, 4-5. In J. Strachey (Ed.), *Standard Edition of the Complete Psychological Works of Sigmund Freud,*

24 volumes. London: Hogarth Press and The Institute of Psycho-Analysis, 1953-1974.

Freud, S. (1905). *Three Essays on Sexuality. SE*, 7: 123-245.

—— (1908). Character and anal erotism. *SE*, 9: 167-175.

—— (1909). *Notes Upon a Case of Obsessional Neurosis. SE*, 10: 153-318

—— (1911). Formulations on the two principles of mental functioning. *SE*, 12: 213-226.

—— (1911). Recommendations to physicians practicing psychoanalysis. *SE*, 12: 109-120.

—— (1915). *The Unconscious. SE*, 14: 159-215.

—— (1915). Instincts and their Vicissitudes. *SE*, 14: 109-140.

—— (1918). *From the History of an Infantile Neurosis. SE*, 17: 3- 123.

—— (1923). *The Ego and the Id. SE*, 19: 3-66.

—— (1926). *Inhibitions, Symptoms and Anxiety. SE*, 20: 77-175.

Grotstein, J.S. (1977). The psychoanalytic concept of schizophrenia. *Int. J. Psycho-Anal.*, 58: 403-452.

Isaacs, S. (1952). On the nature and function of phantasy. In Klein, M., Heimann, P., Isaacs, S., and Riviere, J. (Eds.), *Developments in Psycho-Analysis.* London: Hogarth Press, pp. 67-121.

Joseph, B. (1982). The addiction to near death. *Int. J. Psycho-Anal.*, 63: 449-456.

Kafka, F. (1937). *The Trial.* New York: Alfred A. Knopf.

—— (1948). *The Penal Colony. Stories and Short Pieces.* New York: Schocken Books.

Kandel, E.R. (1991). *Principles of Neural Science.* Chapters 56-57, 62. New York: Appleton and Lange.

—— (1995). *Essentials of Neural Science.* New York: Appleton and Lange.

Klein, M. (1923). Early analysis. In *The Writing of Melanie Klein, 1921-1945.* London: Hogarth Press, pp. 77-105.

—— (1929). Personification in the play of children. In *Contributions to Psycho-Analysis, 1921-1945.* London: Hogarth Press, pp. 215-226.

—— (1933). The early development of conscience in the child. In *Contributions to Psycho-Analysis 1921-1945.* London: Hogarth Press pp. 267-277.

—— (1952). Notes on some schizoid mechanisms. In Klein, M., Heinemann, P., Isaacs, S., and Riviere, J. (Eds.). *Developments in Psycho-Analysis.* London: Hogarth Press, pp. 292-320.

—— (1952). Some theoretical conclusions regarding the emotional life of the infant. In *Developments in Psycho-Analysis.* London: Hogarth Press, pp. 198-199.

—— (1957). *Envy and Gratitude: A Study of Unconscious Sources.* London: Tavistock Pubns.

—— (1961). *Narrative of a Child Analysis.* London: Hogarth Press.

Lemberger, L., Axelrod, J., and Kopin, I.J. (1972). Metabolism and disposition of tetra-hydrocannabinols in naive subjects and chronic marijuana users.

Proc. N.Y. Acad. Sci., 191.

Lyons, J. (1972). Human language. In Hinde, R.A. (Ed.), *Non Verbal Communication.* Cambridge University Press.

Mahler, M. (1968). *On Human Symbiosis and The Vicissitudes of Individuation*, Volume I. *Infantile Psychosis.* New York: Int. Univ. Press.

Mancia, M. (1981). On the beginning of mental life in the foetus. *Int. J. Psycho-Anal.*, 62: 351-355.

Meltzer, D. (1956). Anal omnipotence and projective identification. *Int. J. Psycho-Anal.*, 47.

—— (1967). *The Psycho-AnalyticalProcess.* London: Heinemann.

—— (1973). *Sexual States of Mind.* Perthshire, Scotland: Clunie Press.

—— (1984). *Dream-Life.* Perthshire, Scotland: Clunie Press.

—— (1994). Sincerity: A study in the atmosphere of human relations. In Hahn, A. (Ed.), *Sincerity and Other Works: Collected Papers of Donald Meltzer.* London: Karnac Books, pp. 185-284.

Meltzer, D., Brenner, J., Hoxter, S., Wedell, H., and Wittenberg, I. (1975). *Explorations in Autism.* Perthshire, Scotland: Clunie Press.

Onions, C.T. (Ed.) (1964). *The Shorter Oxford English Dictionary*, 3rd Revised Edition. London: Oxford University Press.

Paul, M.I., Cramer, H., and Bunney, W.E. (1971). Urinary adenosine 3'5' monophosphate in the switch process from depression to mania. *Science*, 171: 300-303.

Paul, M.I. and Carson, I.M. (1976). The sense of strangeness. *Int. Rev. Psycho-Anal.*, 3: 435-440.

—— (1980). A contribution to the study of dimension. *Int. Rev. Psycho-Anal.*, 7: 101-111.

—— (1997). II. Transformational aspects of phantasy under the influence of marijuana. *J. M. Klein Obj. Rel.*, 15(2): 195-212.

Paul, M.I. (1981). A mental atlas of the process of psychological birth. In Grotstein, J.S. (Ed.), *Do I Dare Disturb the Universe? A Memorial to Wilfred R. Bion.* Beverly Hills: Caesura Press, pp. 552-570.

—— (1984). Instrument building in psychoanalysis. Unpublished manuscript.

—— (1989). Notes on the primordial development of the penitential transference. *M. Klein Obj. Rel.*, 7(2): 43-69.

—— (1989). Intonational elements as communication in psychoanalysis. *Free Assns.*, 15: 67-86.

—— (1990). Studies on the phenomenology of mental pressure. *M. Klein Obj. Rel.*, 8(2): 7-29.

—— (1993). A consideration of practical psychoanalytic epistemology. *M. Klein Obj. Rel.*, 11(2): 11-29.

—— (1997). On the imitation of human speech. *J. M. Klein Obj. Rel.*, 15(1): 51-76.

—— (1997). The effects of marijuana on the phenomenology of communication in two-person groups: I. The questionnaire study on subjective experience, *J. M. Klein Obj. Rel.*, 15(2): 179-193.

Piontelli, A. (1986). *Backwards in Time*. Perthshire, Scotland: Clunie Press

—— (1987). Infant observation from before birth. *Int. J. Psycho-Anal.*, 68: 453-463.

—— (1988). Pre-natal life and birth reflected in the analysis of a 2-year-old psychotic girl. *Int. Rev. Psycho-Anal.*, 15: 73-81.

—— (1992). *From Foetus to Child: An Observational and Psychoanalytic Study.* London: Routledge, Chapman and Hall.

Ploye, P.M. (1973). Does prenatal mental life exist? *Int. J. Psycho-Anal.*, 54: 241-246.

Pound, E. (1968). How to read. In Eliot, T.S. (Ed.), *Literary Essays of Ezra Pound.* New York: New Directions.

Rank, O. (1929). *The Trauma of Birth.* London: Routledge and Kegal Paul, Ltd.

Rascovsky, A. (1960). *El Psiquismo Fetal.* PAIDOS: Buenos Aires.

Rosenfeld, H. Personal communication.

Sambamoorthy, P. (1975). *South Indian Music, Book IV.* 4th Ed. Madras: Indian Music Publishing, pp. 176-181.

Segal, H. (1956). Notes on symbol formation. *Int. J. Psycho-Anal.*, 391-397.

Tart, C.T. (1972). States of consciousness and state-specific sciences. *Science*, 176.

Tausk, V. (1919). On the origin of the "influencing machine" in schizophrenia. *Psychoanal. Q.*, 1933, 2(3-4): 519-556.

Tronick, E., et al. (1978). The infant's response to entrapment between contradictory messages in face-to-face interaction. *J. Child Psychia.*, 17(1): 1-3.

Tustin, F. (1981). Psychological birth and psychological catastrophe. In *Autistic States in Children.* London: Routledge, pp. 78-94.

Virgil (1887). *The Aeneid.* Translated by John Dryden, 3rd Ed. London and New York.

Winnicott, D.W. (1949). Birth memories, birth trauma, and anxiety. In *Collected Papers: Through Paediatrics to Psycho-Analysis.* London: Tavistock Pubns., pp. 174-193.

Index

Addiction: alcohol, 61; (near) death, 143; drug, 72; mind-set, 171, 180; misery, 143; phantasy, 175; pressure, 115
Agoraphobia, 24
Alcohol, 73, 89; addiction results, 60; rapid absorption, 156
Amniotic: bag of waters, 125; fluid, 69; membranes, 69
Amphetamine, 73
Amplifier, 52: of mental process, 209
Anal: mode, 199-202; origin, 205; zone, 199
Anatomization of primitive elements, 85
Anxiety, 31, 37, 54, 56, 60, 70, 73, 83, 99, 153, 191, 193, 195, 196, 197, 201, 202, 204, 205, 207, 208, 209; intense, 24, 34, 53, 55, 61, 64, 70, 87, 89, 103-104, 110, 118, 127, 144, 174, 176, 177, 179, 196, 197, 198, 199, 204, 205, 207; and countertransference, 191; and depression, 56; extinction, 201, 202, 204; nameless, 89; "oral", 201; persecutory, 49, 200; phobic, 82; and pressure, 117, 121; primary, 72; protoenvy and, 197, 203-204; and sadness, 170; separation, 64, 125, 177, 199, 208; and symptom formation, 59; theory of, 59;
Argyle, M., 149
Attunement, 150
Autism, 55, 71, 158, 166, 167, 171; Meltzer's subclinical, 167
Autistic: barrier, 173, 179, 190; mechanisms, 158; protection, 22; self-stimulatory mode, 158; states, 120; stimulation, 152
Axelrod, J., 156, 193, 195

Badness, 111
Barbiturates, 73
Beckmann, M., 90
Beethoven, L. v., 146
Biological: clock, 85; forms, 25; inborn awareness of, 202; structures, 19
Bion, W.R., 18-20, 22, 23, 24, 28, 39, 76, 77, 85, 124, 129, 132, 136, 142, 167, 187-189, 203-207; *Attention and Interpretation* (1970), 62, 168, 169; (1975), 24, 70; *Elements of Psycho-Analysis* (1963), 76; formulation of beta element, 207; "Language and the schizophrenic" (1955), 22, 150, 189-191; *Learning from Experience* (1962), 37, 40, 41, 104, 132, 135, 142; legacy, 18, 20; psychoanalytic extensions of Freud, 119; *Second Thoughts* (1967), 40, 54, 71, 99, 205; terms, 63; *Transformations* (1965), 108; (1975), 24, 70; use of imaginative conjecture, 86
Birth: canal, 74; experience, 67, 119; phenomena, 85; process, 25, 59, 172; trauma, 59
Blood: -brain barrier, 156; flow, 70; supply, 73, 74
Brazelton T.B., 145

Bunney, W. E., 120

Cannabis sativa, 156, 193; *see* Marijuana
Caper, R., 191
Carson, I.M., 22, 28, 40, 48, 66, 70, 121, 177
Catatonia, 152
Catecholamine: groups, 120; theory of mood, 120
Chemical: event, 157; substance, 73; trigger, 120
Chomsky, N., 72
Column 2 element, 168, 178; emotion, 168
Communication: analytic, 161; concrete, 181; difficulties, 86; dyadic, 28; of information, 150; interactional, 159; intonational aspects of, 21, 145; link, 86; mental, 99; musical, 147; process, 149; sensory, 177; system, 147; velocity of, 88, 159; vocal, 145, 161
Concrete: bunker, 181; quality, 179; reaction, 157; reference, 101; representation of symbol, 201; rigidity, 179; separation, 36; significance, 32; thinking, 203; way, 184
Condon, W., 145
Conflict, 95, 126; coping with, 195; eating and breathing, 25; ego and id, 187; endopsychic, 188; hostility and reality, 188; Oedipus, 84
Countertransference, 188, 195; anxiety in, 203; apparent vs. authentic location, 188; and "drugging numbness", 148; quasi frustration and indifference, 143

Dante, A., 115
Davis, M., 153
Deadness, 22, 39, 115, 180
Death: experience, 209; instinct, 83, 86
Dedimensionalization, 22
Defense(ive): 199; explosion, 190; maneuvers, 170, 198; posture, 199
Depression, 99; anxieties, 99, 204; experience, 102; feelings, 50; states, 119; *see* Position
Desymbolization, 98, 202
Development: embryologic, 85; libidinal, 85
Dimensionalization: 22, 39; of experience, 39, 40; of parental representations, 48
Domain: of experience, 20, 140; of hallucinatory transformations, 169; of sensory apparatus, 36; of subject, 55
Draconian: code, 26; conscience, 106; elements of judgement, 106
Dream: quasi wakeful states, 94; text, 184; thoughts, 203
Drug: action, 193; activity, 73; addiction, 78; dependency, 78, 79; effect, 195, 201; experience, 201; habituation, 60; -like effects, 22; -tissue interaction, 156; *see* Addiction
Dysphoria, 115; state, 64, 68

Ego: castration of, 189; conflict 85, 187, 189, 203; development, 84; excessive tension in, 83; functions, 189; psychology, 85; and symbol formation, 203;
Eisenberg, R.B., 158
Emotion(al): contact, 41, 99, 130, 170; experience, 37, 104, 206; explosion, 67; link, 119; mind, 175; pain, 60; realization of facts, 191; state, 166; storms, 191; tension, 172; tone, 171; tricks, 172
Envy: 54, 105, 174, 195, 199, 200, 201, 202, 207, 208; Bion's con-

ception of, 142, 168; definition, 105, 297, 209; -in-the-field, 196-197, 199; *See* protoenvy
Enzyme, 77
Epinephrine, 104
Epistemology: practical psychoanalytic, 27, 129-145
Equilibria: mental, 203
Erikson, E., 199
Evacuative control, 201
Evans, B., 146
Exciters: sexual, 141, 142
Excrements, 72
Excretory modes, 50
Externalization, 86

Fetal: activity, 24; aspect of mind, 75; mind, 80; body, 121; circulation, 73; clock, 85; derivation, 75; development, 75; engagement, 86; experience, 75; growth, 85; level, 25, 75, 76; mental set, 75; mind, 23, 86; movement, 24, 85; organization, 104; physiological rhythms, 86; pressure level, 76; sense organization, 85; state of mind, 23
Fetus: 24, 59, 69-72, 85, 86, 104, 116, 119
Freud, S., 19, 59, 82, 83, 85, 105, 112, 113, 147, 148, 187, 188, 189, 190; *A Case of Obsessional Neurosis* (1909), 87; "Character and anal erotism" (1908), 32; "Formulations Regarding Two Principles of Mental Functioning" (1911), 169, 188; *Instincts and their Vicissitudes* (1915), 39, 85; *Interpretation of Dreams* (1900), 36; *Inhibitions, Symptoms and Anxiety* (1926), 60, 85; *The Ego and the Id* (1923), 85; (1924), 187, 199

Galactic void of mental space: infinite, 63
Gap: and anxiety, 196, 199, 209; awareness of, 196, 202, 209; coping with, 202, 204, 208; definition, 196-199; denial of, 198, 204, 209; experience of, 64, 161, 201; perception of, 197, 198, 203, 205, 207, 208, 209; primitive and symbolic language, 72, 204, 209; reality and expectation, 34; self and object, 35, 105, 196, 201, 204
Genital: modes, 199; phase, 84; phenomenon, 48
Genitality, 84
Grammar: depth, 150
Greed, 115, 201; phenotype, 25; excessive, 68; definition, 124, 131, 132
Grotstein, J.S., 23, 24, 27, 42, 97
Grove, R., 147

Hallucination, 20, 40, 169, 186
Hallucinogen, 73, 156
Hallucinosis, 169, 170

Imagoes, 82, 84
Indolamines, 120
Inducers, 165; of replicable experience, 178
Induction of mental pressure, 121
Infant: research, 145; state of mind, 157; vocalizations, 46
Infantile: anxieties, 63; dependency situations, 46; maternal transference, 57, 78; oral phantasies, 24; primitive experiences, 46; relation, 135; sounds, 185; state of pain, 174;
Integration: of data, 36, 37, 207; -dis integration, 20; of mental object, 37; of vision, 36
Intelligence, 102
Interaction(al): group, 196; matrix, 196

Interactive: effects of types of interpretation, 19, 22; mind, 19; patterns of sound, 22; process, 145; relation, 145
Intonation(al): chemical effect of, 157, 158; elements, 145, 155; patterns, 159; prosodic drugs, 170
Intoxication, 194, 195, 199, 201; drug, 193
Intrapsychic: action of defense, 83; induction of mental pressure, 123
Intrauterine: experience, 70; state, 72
Introjection; of good objects, 116; mechanisms, 72; of values, 82; re-introjection, 88
Isaacs, S., 178, 190

Jamal, A., 153
Jealousy, 48, 95, 182; excessive, 46, 120; experience of, 54; as motive force, 46; possessive, 120; primitive, 46; sexualization of, 118
Joseph, B., 143

Kafka, F., 88, 100
Kandel, E.R., 19
Klein, M., 20, 26, 76, 81, 82, 84, 85, 86, 103, 112, 119, 178, 179, 188, 189, 197, 198, 208; *Envy and Gratitude* (1957), 34, 61, 197, 198; "Infant analysis" (1923), 85; *Narrative of a Child Analysis* (1961), 72; "Notes on some schizoid mechanisms" (1946), 108; "Personification in the play of children" (1929), 84; "Some theoretical conclusions regarding the emotional life of the infant" (1952), 72, 79; "The early development of conscience in the child" (1933), 82, 83, 85; "The importance of symbol-formation in the development of the ego" (1930), 189, 191
Kopin, I.J., 156, 193, 195
Korsakoff's psychosis, 187

Language: form, 145, 159; of true effect, 191; structure, 149
Learning process, 28
Lemberger, L., 156, 193, 195
Libido, 59, 83, 85; impulse, 83
Linguistic, 137; considerations, 148; evolution, 32; field, 150; forms; 48; usage, 64, 70
Loneliness, 18, 142
Los Angeles Psychoanalytic Society, 77
Lyons, J. (1972), 148
Lysis: of barrier, 166, 186; of barrier results, 166; of encapsulated autistic state, 165; of pain, 165

Mahler, M., 72
Maintenance of: abstract use of speech, 49; analytic process, 103; of barrier, 173; of continuity of thought, 187; of hermetic seal, 100; jaillike internal world, 100; of performance of task, 115; of pressure, 126; of virtual world, 173
Mancia, M., 85
Manic: defenses, 159; march, 139; style, 123
Marijuana, 28, 193-195, 198, 200, 204, 209; administration, 193; experience, 209; influence of, 28, 193; use of, 196; *see Cannabis sativa*
Marital: difficulties, 129, 133, 150
Masturbation, mental, 181; phantasies, 173
Meltzer, D., 57, 99, 100, 120, 167, 128, 129, 163, 177; *Dream-Life* (1984), 149, 150; *Explorations in Autism* (1975), 40, 55, 167; *Sexual States of Mind* (1973), 101; *The Psycho-Analytical Process* (1967),

34, 109
Memory: acting, 104; of birth process, 109, 120; of deadly quality of mother's voice, 152; retrieval, 47, 50, 57; retrieval system, 48; system, 48
Mental: absence, 108, 109; activity, 84; anatomy, 17; apparatus, 4, 189; atlas, 23, 59; attack, 55; burn, 52; capacities, 34; changes, 147; confusion, 34, 35; contact, 118; coordinates, 17, 108; detritus, 168; development, 23, 85, 142; drugs, 141, 157; effect, 146, 157, 178, 193; events, 68, 182; experience, 27, 36, 160, 176; fact, 132; force, 74; growth, 168; health, 63; journey, 173; language, 116; location, 27, 37, 79, 99; movement, 37, 107, 109; murder, 57; myopia, 57; object, 37, 40; obstruction, 111; operation, 18, 23, 179; organization, 22; pain, 60, 81, 86, 87, 108, 113, 115, 122, 124, 155, 157, 160, 176; phenomena, 86; pressure, 27, 108, 109; process, 20, 23, 24, 29, 73, 75, 132, 134; realm, 108; regulation, 158; representation of gap, 208, 209; retreat, 109; sectors, 126; sense receptors, 146; set, 147, 158, 195; space, 37, 107, 118, 119, 195, 208; state, 35, 36, 64, 176; strength, 141; structures, 17; system, 50; torture, 81, 89; world, 85, 101
Milk, 200, 202
Mimesis, 167; mimetic activity, 179; communication, 190
Mindlessness, 78, 79
Mnemic: image, 59; residues, 23, 59, 76, 101, 103, 104; symbols, 59
Morpheme, 150
Motor: action, 190; discharge, 189
Musical: accompaniment, 159, 160; aspects, 150; elements, 150, 151; forms, 157; notation, 22, 149, 161; patterns, 149
Mutual: participation, 147; suffering, 103

Narcosis, 60, 73, 77
Narcotic diminisher, 142
Negative: connotation, 64; maternal relationship, 78, 78; response, 180; therapeutic reaction, 81, 184
Negativity, 135
Nervous system, 19, 116, 156, 193; parasympathetic, 197
Neuronal: code, 19; structure, 19
Neurosis, 187; obsessional, 105

Object: absent, 202; awareness of, 36, 42, 46; bad, 203; Bion on, 188, 203, 206, 207; damage to, 140, 191; desired, 56; ego and, 203; envy of, 168; external, 57, 83, 194, 208; Freud on, 83, 85; fusion with, 48; good, 116, 203; ideal, 204; internal, 194, 200; lost, 209; maternal, 41, 72; mental, 36, 37, 40, 57; nourishing, 46, 64, 71, 199, 201, 202; omnipotent, 50; part, 36; paternal, 23, 42; phantasy of being inside, 22, 33, 34, 40, 118; placental, 71; possession of, 72; primary, 22, 56; real, 82; regulating, 158; relations, 72, 86, 119, 128-129, 136, 142, 145, 158, 165, 172, 175; representation, 36, 40, 41, 57, 198; self and, 34, 35, 48, 158, 204, 206; separation from, 36, 56, 71, 158; split, 189; subject and, 47, 48; superior, 142; transference, 108; whole, 36, 167
Obscuration: 29, 34, 36
Obsessional, 86, 87, 129; ideas, 87, 88; qualities, 120; states of mind, 81; subclinical form, 166; thinking, 60;

thought, 25, 131
Oceanic bliss, 73
Oedipal: conflict, 84; murder, 55; myth, 55, 57, 76; situation, 57
Oneness, 48
Onions, C.T.: *see Oxford English Dictionary*
Orality, 199, 200
Oxford English Dictionary, 21, 74, 121, 134, 136, 148

Pain: of absence of fulfillment of desires, 168; of absence of need-fulfilling objects' attention, 46; of band-like pressure quality, 66; of experience of first voice, 155; threshold, 158; -inducing phenomenon, 46; -reducing features of sound, 158
Paralinguistic: features, 148, 149; features of language, 149; signals, 149
Paranoid-schizoid: homologue of, 103; states, 119; *see* Position
Parent(al): contact, 46; intercourse, 40, 48, 57; link, 53; object, 42; pair, 46; relationship substitute, 46; representation, 42, 47, 48; sense, 47, 53, 56; sensory modalities, 48; split intercourse, 52
Parricide, 55, 56, 57
Parturition, 69, 104
Paul, M.I., 40, 48, 64, 66, 70, 73, 85, 108, 114, 119, 120, 121, 141, 144, 172, 173, 177, 178
Penis, 53; psychoanalytic, 54
Perceptual: apparatus, 29, 193; organ, 36
Persecutory, 160; anxiety, 49, 200; delusions, 29; experience, 179, 205; ideation, 90
Personality: mutilation of, 174
Personification, 84, 85
Phanopoeia, 146
Phantasied: absent object, 202; contact, 201; feces, 202; invasion, 205; onslaughts, 72; state, 165
Phantasy, 21, 22, 27, 28, 33, 34, 36, 37, 39, 40, 42, 44, 50-52, 54-57, 59, 61, 63, 64, 65, 66, 67, 70-72, 73, 74, 75, 78, 81, 82, 84, 85, 99, 101, 105, 106, 108, 128, 129, 133, 136, 142, 160, 166, 171, 173, 174, 176-180, 182, 193-195, 198-202, 208, 209; of ability, 63; addictive virtual, 174, 175; anal defensive system, 200; of birth process, 66; of crashes, 89; of death, 106; dream-like, 101; Dracula, 73; of drug effectiveness, 200; elements, 79; /expectation, 169; of expulsion, 40; of fusion, 67; of hermetic seal, 167, 190; of imprisonment, 81; interactive, 28; of intercourse, 22, 40; of internal object, 194; maintenance of, 175; of penitence, 81; of prediction, 99; prenatal, 23, 165, 179; of primitive conscience, 118; of punishment, 83, 85, 123; of seal, 118; sensory, 182; segment, 201; sequence, 150; shift, 57; structure, 171, 173; of violent accidents, 69
Pharmacopoeia, 21, 152, 159
Phenomenology, 37, 107, 120, 127, 153; description, 142; experience, 111; of mental pressure, 107-127; psychoanalytic, 18, 25
Phonetics, 148
Phonology, 148, 150
Physical: elements, 156; facts, 132; gap, 208; instability, 132; movement, 108; quality, 66; sensation, 66, 201; substances, 28; violence, 60
Physiology, 65, 59; adaptation, 69
Piontelli, A., 23, 24, 25, 119, 120, 124
Placenta, 70-74; placental barrier, 104;

connection, 74; feed, 64
Plato's dialogues, 160
Ploye, P.M., 76
Pornography, 129, 157; film, 53
Position: 45, 67, 87, 92, 97, 142, 176; depressive, 20, 100, 127, 167, 174, 188, 189, 191; in mental space, 34, 37; paranoid-schizoid, 100, 103, 127
Postnatal: 107; development, 119; experience, 25, 69; influences, 23; state, 86, 119; world, 60
Pound, E., 146
Pregenital: instinctual impulse, 84; states, 84
Prenatal: *anlagen* of superego, 81; epochs, 25; experience, 24, 27, 105; influences, 23, 86; mental world, 107, 109; orientation, 26; pressure, 27; state, 78, 79, 119, 120, 123, 166; transference, 105, 107; world, 117
Primal: identifications, 84; scene, 22, 48, 187
Primeval: mnemic residues, 60; traumatic experiences, 59
Procrastination, 115, 121
Projective identification, 22, 29, 31-35, 51, 61, 65, 73, 75, 77, 100, 109, 179, 198, 203, 205, 208; geography of, 109; Kleinian theory of, 198; maternal-fetal forms, 24; mechanism of, 204; phenomena, 88; results, 205; states, 65
Prosodic: changes, 158; elements of language, 21; features, 148, 149; mechanisms, 160; sequence, 157; signals, 149
Protoenvy: 197, 198, 202-205, 207-209; *see* Envy
Psyche, 83, 207, 220; state of anxiety, 197
Psychic: activity, 88, 104, 112; attachment, 71; birth process, 100; change trigger, 141; closure, 61; experience, 174; field, 108; forward progress, 99; fusion, 21, 32, 48, 56, 57, 65, 90; locale, 36, 37, 49; movement, 24-26, 37, 56, 70, 81, 98, 101, 104, 127, 141, 190; pain, 17, 46, 52, 75, 76, 87, 99, 103, 109, 116, 174, 177, 179, 191; sources, 207; space, 66, 100, 108, 111, 139; states, 23, 24; structure, 99
Psychoanalysis, 17, 18, 21, 23, 101, 108, 120, 129, 132, 136, 139, 141, 145, 150, 158, 161, 172, 174; of pregnancy, 24
Psychoanalytic: approach, 173; context, 24, 195; evidence, 63; interpretation, 18; method, 209; process, 51, 81, 113, 128; reception apparatus, 19; research, 79; session, 40, 47, 120; setting, 147; tactics, 172; technique, 156; theory, 22, 105; tool, 129; transformations, 20; venture, 20; verbal intercourse, 170; work, 20, 28, 180
Psychological: birth, 59, 64, 70, 120; differentiation, 56; effects, 193; effects of sound density, 153; interpretation of data, 193; interpretation of primary autonomic phenomena, 193; pain, 196; point of view, 194; structure, 149; turbulence, 76
Psychology, 59
Psychopathology, 101, 158
Psychosis, 156, 187, 189, 190, 203; *see* Psychotic
Psychosomatic: considerations, 193; defensive functions, 200; excuses, 132; experience, 204, 209; illness, 116; phantasized defense, 202
Psychotic: parents, 179; part of personality, 123, 124, 136, 142, 144; rage, 124; state, 167, 204

Rank, O., 59
Rascovsky, A., 76
Rat Man, 87
Rectum, 200
Religion, 107
Replicability, 17, 112, 136, 156, 166, 173, 178
Representation of: audition, 47; of change, 37; concrete, 203; emotional experience, 220; of gap, 209; of object, 36; of parent, 34; of parental couple, 46; of prenatal experience, 60, 64; of time, 205
Rosenfeld, H., 159

Sadomasochism, 25, 143
Sander, L.W., 145
Schizophrenia, 189, 190
"Seducers," 141, 142, 153, 157
Segal, H.: "Notes on symbol formation" (1956), 72, 203-204
Sensory: actuality, 204; apparatus, 204; deprivation, 204, 207; experience, 119, 208; information, 39; input, 70; integrative experience, 57; mode, 39; organizational links, 47; organizational pattern, 47; representations, 40, 57; systems, 37
Sensous, 119, 129, 168, 180; experience, 201, 202, 209; feeling, 201; form, 201; interchange, 175; origin, 129; pleasure, 120; qualities, 120; world, 129
Sexual: act, 87, 52, 129; purpose, 118; sensations, 104, 172
Sexualization of pressure, 118
Shambamoorthy, P., 156
Signifier: of state of stupor, 35; of zero coordinate, 111
Simile, 150
Socrates, 160
Soma, 72, 207
Somatic, 116; connection, 207; experiential language, 72; localization, 207; sources, 207
Speech: rhythm of, 159; interactions, 145; pattern, 66; stilted form of, 49; velocity, 56, 139, 160
Stereotype, 145, 166, 173
Strauss, R., 146
Stravinsky, I., 146
Superego: archaic, 26, 81, 82, 95, 88, 99, 100, 141, 142, 143, 144, 173; Bion's notion, 142; dating, 27, 85; definition, 82, 105; development, 89, 104, 119; elements, 26, 50, 102; envious, 106; Freud's theory, 85; gating function, 100; in children, 82, 85; Klein's theory, 82-85, 90, 91; prenatal *anlagen*, 81; primordial, 25, 26; sources, 82, 104, 105; structure, 99, 100, 107
Synchrony, 66

Tausk, V., 143
Therapeutic: alliance, 89; impasse, 81; session, 29; situation, 50
Threeness, 48
Transference: infanticidal, 61; penitential, 81-106; psychotic, 71; situation, 134
Tustin, F., 166, 167
Twoness, 48, 105

UCLA Department of Psychiatry, 28
Uterine: environment, 86; inertia, 69; motility, 104; musculature, 86; pressure, 121; rhythmic contractions, 105; sanctuary, 71; phantasy of u. wall, 100
Uterus, 103

Vergil's *Aeneid*, 77
Visual: acuity, 65; apparatus, 39; channel, 39, 51; clarity, 65; effects, 154; elements, 179; experience, 44,

49, 52; expulsion, 51; encapsulated drugged state, 181; fantasy, 118, 130; free associations, 46; idea, 39; images, 44, 53, 61, 169, 176, 182, 193; information, 40, 53; phantasies, 89, 101, 109, 136, 178, 186, 198; process, 180; production, 181; realm, 51; representation, 39; sense, 55; system, 52; terms, 39-41; thought, 24; version, 51

Vocal: elements, 149; interaction, 52, 145; patterns, 157, 158; qualities, 68; response organization, 145; sound, 152; stimuli, 152

Voice, 147: tone of, 146; force, 67; quality, 149

Washington, N., 128

Weirdness, 36, 37

Winnicott, D.W., 79

Zonal modes, 199, 209